STORIES OF THE OTHER MEDICINE

CURIOSITIES ABOUT IRIDOLOGY AND ACUPUNCTURE

LORENZO MAZZUCCO

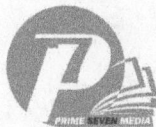

PRIME SEVEN MEDIA

CONTENTS

INTRODUCTION

The first idea for this book was to tell a few stories or anecdotes about unconventional and lesser-known medicine. Then, I also wanted to create a small manual of natural remedies and tips to combat the most common ailments. This is an attempt to merge these two ideas, so that, in the end, it is not a book of stories nor a manual of alternative remedies. However, all things considered, the idea of combining the two, i.e. proposing a remedy and at the same time telling something about its historical source did not seem bad to me. It was important to make known that part of medicine which is less known and today fortunately somewhat revalued. Grandma's remedies always have a special charm and sometimes they still work, even if they have no clear scientific basis and only rely on folk traditions.

So I have collected the many notes I took when I was studying medicine at the University of Florence, in particular at the Master of Integrative Medicine, and I have tried to put them together in an organic manner, to give some suggestions or some help to all those who are skeptical about the traditional methods of classical western medicine, or who are curious to know about some other possibility of treating the most common ailments (insomnia, headaches, joint pain, stress, hypertension, or allergies) without the risk of suffering from the side effects of various drugs.

Topics have been grouped under nutrition, lifestyle, longevity, acupressure, auricular therapy and iridology.

On Iridology

This is a somewhat special topic and is the soul of this book. The analysis of the iris is a very ancient diagnostic method, abandoned by classical medicine for a long time and only recently rediscovered and revalued.

To be in good health, of body and mind, would be a good thing even if rare, especially after a certain age. Normally, those who are well and healthy do not worry so much about their state, behave carefree, eat and drink what they want, go to bed late and easily indulge in a few transgressions. But, when we discover that we have some minor ailment we begin to wonder what, if anything, could have happened and what could be the cause of our discomfort, perhaps we think about what we have eaten, or what we have not done, with our behavior.

The answer could either be that we have overlooked some basic rules of good health or that we have done nothing to prevent the problem. They say prevention is better than cure, but by the time we find the problem, it is already too late. It should have been thought of before!

So this is what iridology can be used for. It fills this curiosity. By analyzing the iris, one can understand, in some cases, the cause of the discomfort or get an idea of the general state of psychophysical health. This book will give you an idea of the potential of this type of investigation, with some examples.

Certainly it is not a rigorous method of investigation, although supported by several studies, it cannot compete with or replace classical and instrumental analyses, however it can give interesting indications that may elude other methods. In some particular cases, such as magnesium deficiency, which cannot be detected by blood tests, it has some advantages. One hears that the iris is the mirror of the soul and thus one can glimpse some tendency or predisposition of the mind.

Back pain.

It all started here! As a young man, I was often afflicted by back pain and so I began to document myself out of curiosity to see what was around, both in literature and on the internet. But what interested me most was the practice, that is, how to really solve the problem. In a more curious fashion, I started practicing Shiatsu and then the Feldenkrais method. Fantastic experiences, all good, very interesting, and also some very good results.

This was not enough for me, of course. I continued to deepen the research on my own. I studied so much that I realized I was prepared enough to try to pass the exam to enter the Faculty of Medicine at the University of Florence. So I got access to the School of Human Health, as the School of Medicine is called today. I started by studying Podiatry, then Osteopathy, and finally Integrative Medicine, with a master in Naturopathy.

In this collection you will find, more or less stated, timid suggestions to fight in different ways the most common discomforts, using the magic of acupuncture points on the body and on the ear and the ability of our body to rebalance the circulating energy and allow a sort of self-healing. I also collected news about the analysis of the iris and the interesting diagnostic indications that can be obtained from careful observation of the eye, with many examples.

Enjoy reading!

Thanks for your comments, observations, and criticisms.

CHAPTER 1

UNCONVENTIONAL MEDICINES

W e often hear about other medicines like alternative and complementary medicine. But there is a bit of confusion; the name itself does not matter, while what is interesting is to understand that it is something different from the official medicine, which is not opposed but flanked. The correct term would be integrative medicine, a set of practices that integrates with classic methods. The terms functional medicine or natural medicine is also widely used. To simplify; it could be said that classical and official medicine is mainly concerned with the symptom and how to treat it, while the other medicine deals with the person as a whole and seeks out the causes of the disorder that can eventually be removed more naturally without the use of chemicals.

The first is also called allopathic medicine, which uses specific drugs at a therapeutic level. The second must devise a strategy based on natural remedies such as physiotherapy, massage, acupressure, and ancient procedures. These remedies were used in the past when there were no drugs, but now they are rediscovered. The first is based on a solid set of data collected from studies and experiments, universally recognized, even if sometimes polluted by some economic interest. On the other hand, the second believes or trusts more in ancient history, tradition, and Grandmother's remedies. Often, it is criticized, precisely, for this scarcity of scientific basis. However, today there are also a lot of scientific data available to confirm its validity.

Acupuncture is considered the first example of integrative medicine, and it is thought to have a history of around 5,000 years. After years of significant results and recognition, finally, in 1979, the World Health Organization (WHO) recognized the effectiveness of this technique in the treatment of 43 diseases. In 2003, the WHO published the official report on the efficacy of acupuncture from controlled clinical trials.

Integrative medicine has been able to re-evaluate ancient methods at the diagnostic level, now in disuse, such as observing the tongue, feeling the pulse, and analyzing the iris.

So, let's see what the advantages of the other medicines are:

They have a lower risk of side effects

- They take advantage of the concept of the natural self-healing of the individual, seen as a global set of the mind, body, and spirit. Chapter 3: Reflexology
- They are less invasive and more economical.
- They encourage knowledge and awareness of the body.
- They manage to solve those problems that conventional methods have been incapable. Thus, they are considered the last resort dictated by desperation.
- It is designed as preventive medicine (see iridology).

Let's see some ways to heal naturally and without drugs.

Acupuncture and Traditional Chinese Medicine
Naturopathy (natural medicine, iridology)
Acupressure
Auricular neuromodulation
Aromatherapy
Phytotherapy
Chromotherapy
Reflexology
Homeopathy
Chiropractic
Osteopathy
Meditation
The massage (Tuinà, shiatzu)
Hypnotherapy
Reiki
Yoga, Qicong
Music therapy.

CURIOSITY ABOUT ACUPUNCTURE

A cupuncture represents, for the Western world, the fulcrum of traditional Chinese medical science. It is an ancient, complex method that involves the stimulation of well-defined points (acupoints) encoded on the body surface, along paths called meridians, through the insertion of thread-like needles, to interact with body homeostasis. It is also to restore a certain energy balance.

The origins:

Although it has been a technique in use for millennia, it has only been scientifically studied in the last twenty-thirty years. It was considered an illegal practice for official medicine only a few decades ago, and some doctors who started practicing it were disqualified from the register. Acupuncture was probably born 3000 or more years ago in response to the need to alleviate suffering and fight diseases with the few means available at that time. Interesting archaeological findings have been found that suggest that the use of needles was known in even more remote times.

What could be the remedies, fashionable at that time, to combat the various and most common ailments? I imagine it could be multiple manipulations, heat compresses, the properties of different herbs or infusions, or other witchcraft. There is a considerable number of stories and anecdotes about its his discovery. One day, a soldier wounded by an arrow reported that he was instantly healed of back pain. This fact started a series of research and studies for a new therapy based on the introduction of needles (see chap 4, the history of the bladder meridian and frozen shoulder)

The emperor, Shen Nung (2700 BC), nicknamed the divine farmer, was one of the first architects of the study of medicine of that time. Many discoveries in the field of botany are due to him. See the chapter 5 on hot water.

A contemporary founding father of acupuncture is the Yellow Emperor, Huang Di, author of the first significant document written, the 'Yellow Emperor's Canon of Internal Medicine.' Many of these insights are still considered valid and applied today.

Diffusion in the West ...

Portuguese and Dutch missionaries in the 16th century

In the sixteenth century, the Portuguese and Dutch missionaries were among the first to bring the novelty of acupuncture from the East. (Jacobus Bontius, a Dutch surgeon, and Hermann Bischoff, a Dutch priest) but these curiosities remained closed in the circle of a few medical enthusiasts. But the diffusion in the West was due to U.S. President Nixon's visit to Chinese Chairman Mao in Beijing , which was a historic event.

Nixon's visit to Mao Tzetung in 1972

It had a significant media effect in the West. This came when a famous New York Times reporter, James Reston, published a curious article in his newspaper about treating his appendicitis with acupuncture in Beijing for post-operative pain.

Mechanism of action

It is thought that health and disease depend on vital energy flow (Qi) along the body and, in particular, along the 12 months where the points are located.

The pain and symptoms of the disease are considered blocking or imbalance of this flow, which can be re-established with pressure, heat, manipulation, and the insertion of needles.

Conclusions: Main effects:

Analgesic
Immune modulator
Deconstructing
Antispasmodic

Anxiolytic

Antidepressant

Many of the mechanisms on which it is based remain unclear. However, there is irrefutable efficacy for various indications such as: Migraine, musculoskeletal pain, tension headache, infertility, anxiety, depression, and insomnia.

In many cases, acupuncture is more effective than conventional drugs.

Several protocols can be found to combat various common problems in the last chapter.

Advantages and disadvantages

The main advantage of acupuncture is that it has no contraindications (except in the state of pregnancy) and has no adverse side effects. It is relatively simple to apply and inexpensive.

A disadvantage is that generally, the public is not so enthusiastic about being pierced with needles; this fact, unfortunately, has limited its widespread use.

Acupuncture without needles.

But alongside acupuncture, acupressure (finger pressure) has developed simultaneously, a simple technique that uses the same principle but without the need for needles obtaining the same results.

Instead of needles, metal spheres or cow seeds can stimulate points or more or less pointed wooden instruments for pressure on specific points.

The use of heat (moxibustion) also exploits the properties of acupuncture points.

The advantage of these procedures, which are not invasive, is that they can also be practiced by non-strictly medical personnel and even experienced by themselves. Even light, colored light, chromo puncture, in some cases, can replace the needle. Today, electrostimulation or laser is also very trendy.

CHAPTER 3

REFLEXOLOGY

Together with acupuncture, there has always been another technique that uses the same principles: Reflexology.

The most famous and most used is the one related to the areas of the foot, but all our body can somehow reflect or communicate with our brain the many information received from the solicitation on the skin, ear, hand, face etc. Later on, we will see in detail, the auricular reflexology and its efects, incredibly.

History of Planter Refloxology

Reflexology has a very ancient history: the first treatments made by massaging the feet were applied in China and India in 5000 BC, where medical therapies were used using finger pressure to influence the body's energy fields (acupuncture, acupressure, shiatsu). Still now, it is widespread in the west.

To testify the antiquity of this practice is the "Tomb of the Doctors" in Saqqara (Egypt, about 2330 BC), where on the walls is painted a scene of massage of the feet and hands. The practice was exported to the West, thanks to the famous Greek doctor called Hippocrates who taught his disciples foot massage.

The practice was used by dentists and when the New York doctor Edwin F. Bowers knew Fitzeralg's technique, he decided to spread reflexology in the United States – thanks to treatises containing the operating principles of Reflexology based on the theories of the Boston doctor.

The method, called "zonal therapy", was centered on pressure carried out both with the hands and with other instruments. The body was divided into ten zones, from the toes to the head, along which energy flows.

Operating Principles

Among the theories that attempt to explain the mechanisms that govern the effectiveness of reflexology, there are, at least, six main ones:

Nerve stimulation

Based on the reaction between the nerve endings present in the reflex zones and the point where the pain is present. The pressure on the reflex zone would then have the task of sending communications to the brain, stimulating it to intervene on the problem encountered.

Release of hormones

Based on the discovery of the brain's control over the endocrine system. According to the theory of reflexology is sufficient to massage the painful reflex zones, to stimulate the brain to release brain hormones, such as endorphin, resulting in therapeutic action.

Stimulation of the lymphatic system

This is favored by the pressure of some reflex points that would implement the acceleration of lymphatic circulation with benefits on the whole body.

Stimulation of the blood system

This aims at improving circulation and decreasing the presence of waste.

Electrical potential

Which would be created between various parts of the body. According to the model of reflexology, the reflex points are comparable to switches while the organs perform the function of accumulators and therefore acting on the switches would reactivate the electrical circulation.

Psychological influences

Explainable by the great importance that the mind has on the origin of physical disorders.

AIRF Italian Association of Reflexologists Federated Acupuncture and reflexology

CHAPTER 4

BACK PAIN AND
MY FROZEN SHOULDER

With the occasion of telling these first stories, I present these three acupuncture points, which are identified by three elements: their name followed by the meridian to which they belong and a progressive number indicating their precise location on the meridian:

Kunlun Bl 60 , Tiaokou ST 38 Chengshan Bl 57

The ancient history of medicine is full of stories, fables, and fascinating legends, verbally handed down in ancient times; often, the stories were fictionalized or magnified as it often happens when stories passed from mouth to mouth from grandparents to grandchildren. However, medical science, supported by numerous scientifically validated studies, is forced to take it seriously.

Antiquity was a period filled with numerous conflicts between various contending groups, perhaps over the possession of a water supply or the ownership of a strategic space. At that time, one of the few weapons available was arrows, in addition to stones, and warriors often returned from battles wounded by these rudimentary points. It seems that the study of this type of wound was responsible for the birth of acupuncture, based on the evidence of the facts. There are a couple of curious legends worth telling. The first story is about a soldier who often complained of severe back pain and could never find a remedy. One day, returning from a battle, wounded by an arrow under the external malleolus, he declared that all his pains had magically disappeared after suffering this wound. Indeed, some doctors of the time become curious and begaan to investigate the properties of these wounds caused by sharp points. Today, we know that particular spot has a specific name, Kunlun (BL-60). This is a point 60 on the bladder meridian.

It is a widely used point, a classic today, for treating lower back pain, headache, and other ailments.

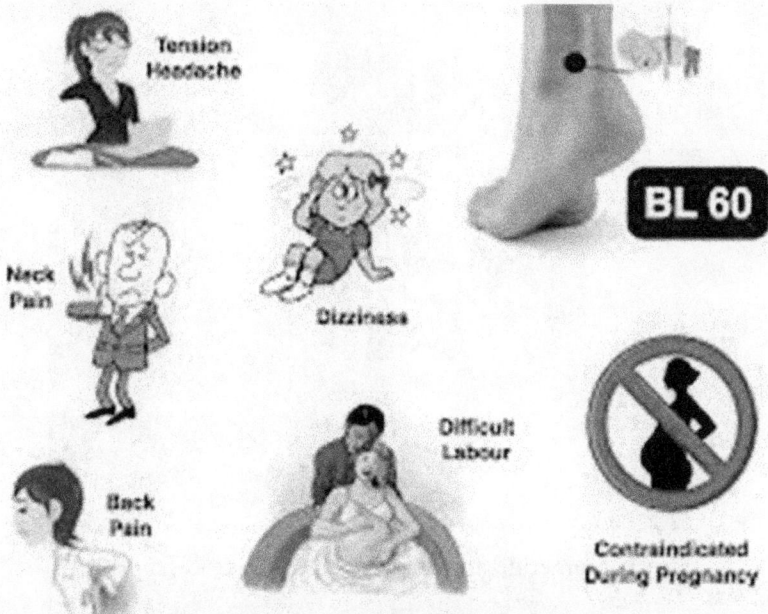

Tension Headache

Neck Pain

Dizziness

BL 60

Back Pain

Difficult Labour

Contraindicated During Pregnancy

In another part of China, perhaps even at different times, the story of another fighter wounded by an arrow is told. The soldier complained of severe pain and limitations in movement in the shoulder area. Today this pathology is well known as "frozen shoulder" or, more appropriately, adhesive capsulitis. . Also, in this case, the medicine of the time could not find any suitable remedy. But one day, the soldier was wounded by an arrow in the center of the leg, and returning to visit his doctor declared that his pain had significantly decreased and then disappeared for good.

The doctor, from that day and successfully began to treat this pathology with the insertion of rudimentary needles.

Today, we know that one of the most used and tested points to treat the frozen shoulder is the Tiaokou ST 38, the point 38 along the stomach meridian, which is located approximately in the center of the leg on the anterior tibialis muscle.

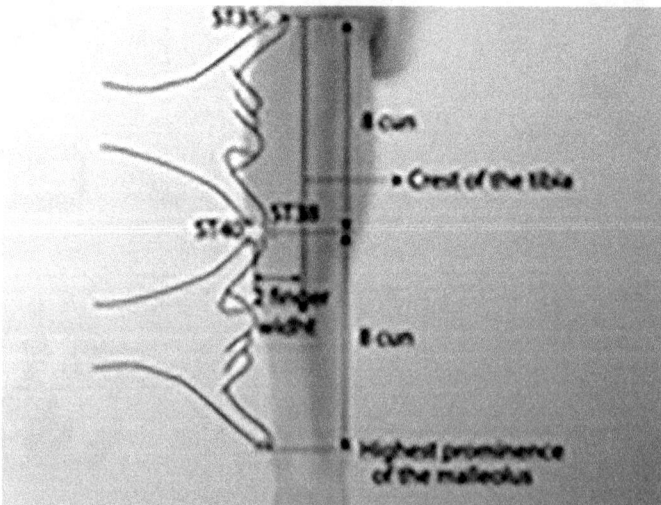

https://acumeridianpoints.com/stomach-st-40-fenglong/

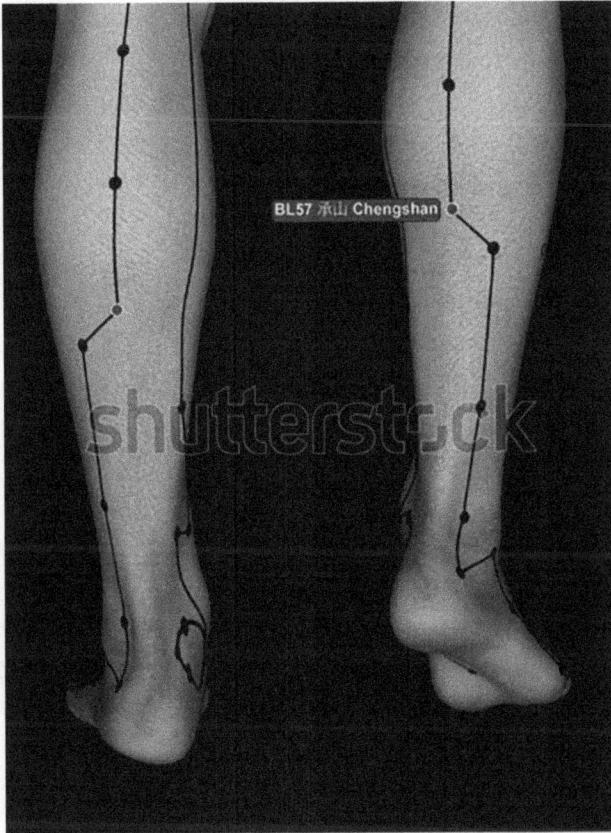

An opposite point, located at the base of the calf, precisely in the center under the two bellies of the gastrocnemius muscle, could also be affected. This is the point BL -57 Chengshan, on the bladder meridian, often cited in the literature as a point of excellent analgesic properties. Probably the arrow crossing the leg has affected both points.

We began to think of a sort of reflexology that must have been quite strange that the solicitation of a point distant from the painful area could alleviate the discomfort. Accepting this fact was undoubtedly a significant step forward.

I want to tell you this story because it happened to me.

I must admit that it is a very annoying disorder and will not allow you to sleep. You are constantly forced to change position to limit that extreme pain. You do not wish anyone to experience this discomfort. Today, in classical medicine, it is possible to intervene with painkillers or physiotherapy practices successfully.

Both solutions did not fascinate me at all, and so I began to investigate, and I discovered that the acupuncture technique, a few thousand years old, was still in vogue. So, I treated my colon with needles, and the disturbance disappeared as if by magic. This cannot be considered a scientific verification because it is a single isolated case that cannot be used as an example. However, in my case, it worked. Maybe I would have healed spontaneously by myself, and perhaps I was just lucky. However, it is a fact, but not the only one.

Returning to my back pain, which was the origin of all these studies of mine, I must say, with some satisfaction, that at the moment, I no longer suffer from it, at least pre-now, thanking both the classic acupuncture on the body and the ear. It will never be known whether the contribution to obtaining this kind of healing is due to a better and careful lifestyle (physical activity, fasting, nutrition), prevention against humidity, or precisely to the magic of acupuncture.

All the stories I tell you always have something magical or imperceptible. Read, out of curiosity, the stories of Dr. Feldenkrais, or those of Dr. Edward Bach (1886-1936), that of flowers. They all have something magical.

CHAPTER 5

THE DISCOVERY OF HOT WATER

D rinking hot water after boiling it is not really a bad idea, even today, in Europe, where the level of hygiene is relatively high, the practice is still esteemed. This precaution is suggested when traveling to Third-World countries. Instead, imagine how the level of hygiene in China in 2700 BC could have been – poverty, malnutrition, various diseases, without a precise idea of medicines and a very high mortality rate, both in childhood and adulthood.

A curiosity: it is said that at that time, Emperor Shen Nung was somewhat disappointed by the situation of too many sick people who were around, and they could not pay taxes. And for this reason, he worked hard to study remedies and encourage various health practices to heal people who thus could not escape the payment of taxes. , today the situation is paradoxically the opposite. The sicker there are, the more economic interests revolve around the problem, and as the famous Doctor Franco Berrino points out, the more health problems there are, GDP increases. There would be some reflection!

However, it seems that thanks to Emperor Shen Nung, drinking hot water was very fashionable in those days. This character, called the divine healer, the great botanist, and the divine farmer, had the merit of being the first to start studying the first possible remedies for the many diseases that his people were confronted with. It seems he had a passion for medical research and delighted in selecting plants, herbs, leaves, and roots. He then worked, treated, and experimented with, sometimes, even on himself and his subjects to evaluate their effect or therapeutic efficacy.

He experimented and catalogued more than three hundred substances derived from botany. Some later revealed to be toxic (about seventy), others with particular therapeutic properties, so he was rightly called the father of Chinese botany.

He was able to describe a hundred remedies that are still valid today. He was the first, for example, to discover the therapeutic effects of cannabis. We also remember ginseng, turmeric, ginger, which are back in fashion today, especially those who love to take care of themselves directly from nature.

There was no trace of all this work at the time; All the exciting discoveries were verbally handed down from generation to generation. Finally and fortunately, after several years, they were collected and published in the Classic on the herb, roots of the divine farmer.

(Only about 2,300 years later, in Greece, a particular famous physician named Hippocrates (Kos, 460 BC - Larissa, 377 BC), the father of our western medicine, began to do more or less the same things that were later published in the Corpus Hippocraticum)

Thus, during these experiments, many patients unfortunately died, many others recovered from some ailment and nothing happened to others. With great care, the emperor noted the results and tried to understand the possible associations. For example, bitter herbs were good for the liver; ginger warmed up, ginseng was aphrodisiac and revitalizing, and so on.

However, during these classifications, he made one of the most exciting discoveries, 'the banalest'. He had divine illumination and realized never got sick among his closest subjects who drank hot water after boiling. In contrast, unlike ordinary people who drank water directly from reserves or wells, he became ill all the time. And so he had the brilliant idea of publishing a document in which it was imposed, throughout China, to drink only hot boiled water.

So, in those days, every house always had to have a pot of hot water. So, it is said that one day the emperor, while he was drinking his classic cup of hot water, sitting under a camellia plant, by chance, a leaf fell into his cup.

The water changed color and also released a specific particular aroma. He, who used to taste everything after drinking it, had such a pleasant and refreshing effect that he was fascinated by it. He wanted to know better than the plant that had produced this leaf, thus favoring its use, study, cultivation, and experimentation.

Hence the birth of tea. An exciting property of tea, which he later discovered, was an effective antidote against many poisonous herbs he was studying.

It is said that once, he was in danger of dying from poisoning from the toxic effects of a poisonous plant. It seems his incredible drink saved him.

He had also discovered the properties of licorice as an antidote to a specific type of poisoning. Even today, licorice is recognized as having beneficial and protective properties for the liver.

Ironically, it is thought that he died of poisoning of a herb he was experimenting with, a herb that breaks the intestine, and was unable to take the antidote in time. However, he died more than a hundred years old.

He remains a character with incredible organizational and creative ability. He is credited with the ideas of producing cereals, the famous five cereals: corn, fenugreek, rice, millet, and oats.

Many years have passed, and today we have rediscovered countless other properties of tea.(Certainly not used as an antidote for poisoning) Green tea is very popular today among wellness enthusiasts, a little different from the standard black tea.

There are many different preparations for this type of tea, especially in Japan. (The most famous is Matcha which is sold in powder form and requires special preparation. Very bitter. However, it has incredible antioxidant power; 100 gr of powder gives about 1750.000 units orac.) It deserves particular attention because it doesn't exist as a healthy drink in the world. It is obtained from the same plant as the classic tea, camellia Sinensis, but with a different, non-fermentative process.

10 Health Benefits of Green Tea

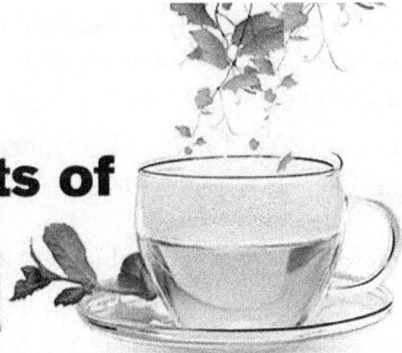

1 Green Tea Fights Off Allergies

10 Green Tea Regulates Your Blood Sugar Levels

9 Green Tea Makes You Happy

2 Green Tea Makes You Smarter

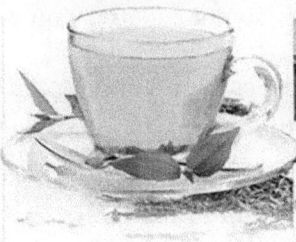

8 Green Tea Lowers Cholesterol

3 Green Tea Makes Your Teeth and Gums Stronger

7 Green Tea Improves Eyesight

4 Green Tea Helps You Live Longer

5 Green Tea Improves Your Skin

6 Burns fat

Healthy Hubb
www.healthyhubb.com

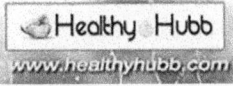

Compared to black tea, it has a much higher content of that particular polyphenol, Epigallocatechingallate the EGCG, considered responsible for its numerous properties such as the anti-inflammatory one inhibits the production of the proinflammatory cytokine TNF-alpha.

Green tea contains flavonoids, catechins, tannins, theophylline, B vitamins, minerals, and amino acids. The properties of green tea are mainly tonic, diuretic, purifying, and antioxidant. It has no particular contraindications, and it is always a drink recommended for a healthy lifestyle, also given the low caffeine content. (a cup of green tea contains 80 to 140 mg of polyphenols and 50 mg of caffeine, about a third of that contained in a cup of coffee).

Some argue about the bitter taste, due to the tannins, limits the large consumption, but it is also true that it is enough to use a water temperature of around 80 degrees instead of 100 to overcome this drawback. In addition to the many excellent properties recently discovered, antioxidants, anti-inflammatory, anticancer, and hypoglycemic can help prostate problems. A 150 ml cup of tea brings about 1,800 Orac units, so not bad as an antioxidant.

The term ORAC, an acronym for Oxygen Radicals Absorbance Capacity (i.e., Absorption Capacity of Oxygen Radicals), indicates the antioxidant capacity of foods, i.e., the ability to fight and eliminate free radicals that are present in our body.

CHAPTER 6

THE CORRECT LIFESTYLE

A set of behaviors and habits to be followed with a certain continuity, within certain rules and recommendations, with the aim of maintaining a good state of health and preventing possible future ailments in time. It is often said that prevention is better than cure.

This could be a definition of proper lifestyle, but let's see what to focus on.

In my opinion, there are four points that we should bear in mind:

- ➲ Healthy eating (possibly fasting)
- ➲ Regular physical activity
- ➲ Improve the quality of sleep
- ➲ Free, purify the mind from all stress techniques of breathing, meditation, relaxation

If we think about bad state of health or illnesses, they often have at the base, as causes, the non-respect of these four points. So one possible recipe for better health could be to engage in proper nutrition, frequent physical activity, better quality sleep and calm the mind. Easy to say. But a great advantage to get great results instead of resorting to the use of drugs.

All drugs carry a lot of side effects that often generate other problems.

The aim of integrative medicine is to avoid the use of various drugs as much as possible. Let's see what to put in the viewfinder to frame the goal of a proper lifestyle.

At the first place, surely, the quality (also the quantity) of food.

Let's see what lessons and insights of wisdom can be gained from studying the history of a few centuries ago. Hippocrates of Kos (460 a. C. circa - m. 370 a. C. circa) was a physician in ancient Greece, considered the father of Western medicine. Among the wonderful insights and discoveries, he argued that food should be the first medicine.

What to eat, what not to eat, when and how much? That is the challenge. The variables are many, the solutions are infinite.

Often family habits, cultural or regional traditions are so deeply rooted in the population that it is difficult to question them and make radical changes.

Weight

Losing weight is a good idea and also undoubtedly healthy. The first rule that always works is that of common sense that is, to eat little and do a regular physical activity. Better, it would be, to keep under control the abdominal circumference, which turns out to be more important than the weight itself. The abdominal circumference, (maximum limit: 80 cm for women and 95 cm for men) is considered an element to be considered as a risk factor, number one, in metabolic syndrome, that is in the prevention of cardiovascular diseases This fat deposit produces highly inflammatory cytokines in addition to other considerable damage.

Optimal Feeding Behavior

When I studied Integrative Medicine at the University of Florence, optimal feeding behavior was a highly discussed topic and open to many hypotheses and interpretations. But the central point was to define the most important characteristics of nutrients for good overall prevention and maybe delay aging.

They are three simple concepts. Nutrients should be first of all:

AAA-----Anti-inflammatory Anti-oxidants Anti-acid

Anti-inflammatory

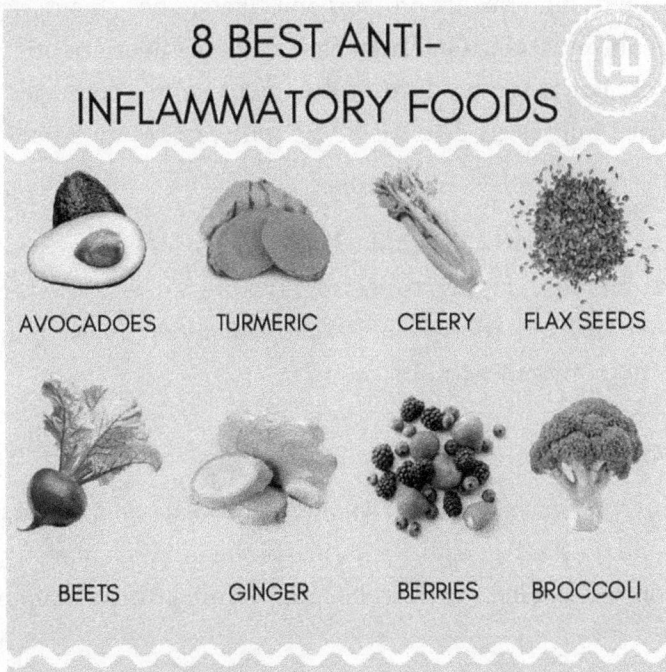

https://www.mealfit.co/

29

Inflammation?

Consider the two forms of inflammation; acute and chronic.

Acute inflammation is a natural protective mechanism for our body, a normal response to every kind of diseases, injuries, and anything it considers harmful. In general, it is a positive, temporary action that helps the immune system to defend us, until this state lasts over time and becomes chronic then it becomes negative. Although chronic inflammation is low-level and often silent, the damage it can cause is varied, with many possible complications.

Foods and supplement that fight inflammation: Omega-3 Fatty Acids: Salmon, Tuna, sardines; Seeds and Dried Fruit

Oilseeds, are a mine of nutritional and healthy properties. They are an excellent source of antioxidants, anti-inflammatory, minerals, vitamins, omega 3 fats, high quality proteins and fibers. They should never be missing on our table. They also have a remarkable satiating power and fortunately their production does not require special industrial treatments. Suggested dose 20-30 gr. (one or two tablespoons) but beware of calories.

These are really better than a medicine! Great for cholesterol, blood pressure, blood sugar, heart disease. Hydrophilic properties, induce satiety, antioxidants (polyphenols), anti-inflammatory. Rich in fiber, magnesium, manganese and omega 3.

Flaxseed

Excellent for reducing pressure, cholesterol, blood sugar, risk of cancer (breast and prostate) and also intestinal problems. Rich in manganese, magnesium, thiamine (vitamin B1) iron . Anti-inflammatory omega 3.

The nuts are excellent for their many healthy properties, they contain polyunsaturated fats, alpha-linoleic acid of the omega 3 family. Beware, because they also contain many omega 6 and should not be abused, because they are pro-inflammatory. Nuts also contain melatonin, so they are great for better sleep and are also good for diabetics.

They give energy, improve brain functions, rich in magnesium and potassium, lower cholesterol and regulate pressure

Spices: Ginger / Turmeric

Ginger

Ginger, is the root of a perennial herbaceous plant belonging to the Zinziberacee family. A spice considered, anciently, miraculous for its properties: digestive, diuretic, anti-inflammatory, antibacterial, painkillers, hypoglycemic and also aphrodisiac. Excellent source of potassium (415 mg).

Turmeric is a spice known for its bright golden yellow color (Curcuma longa), belonging to the same family as Ginger. Together they are part of the mixture of spices that make up Indian curry. It prevents and reduces inflammation, a natural painkiller, protects the liver, aids digestion, limits the action of free radicals, strengthens the immune system. It has a low bioavailability so it should be consumed together with black pepper. es.

Avocado

It's the perfect nutrient! It does not lack anything, excellent source of omega 3 fats, it also has an excellent satiating power. It, thus, improves digestion, relieves joint pain and constipation, and regulates pressure. It also improves eyesight, lowers cholesterol, improves skin and hair health

Berries

It's a generic term that includes a series of small fruits with very interesting properties. Unfortunately, majority of those on the market did not grow naturally in the woods. It would be ideal to collect them in person when they are in season, because they contain about twice as many vitamins and other minerals. Good idea to freeze them, once purchased fresh. In general, they are excellent antioxidants, anti-inflammatory, rich in vitamins, fiber and mineral salts. They regulate pressure, cholesterol; improve memory an delays cellular aging.

Blueberry (vaccinium myrtillus).

They are located in the mountains, because they prefer the cold. They improve vision, indicated for microcirculation disorders, prevent the damage of diabetes, hypertensive retinopathy. They are rich in vit C and vit A , mineral salts (Na, K, Ca, Fe, Ph) and fibers (3.1 gr). Anthocyanins, which give the color purple black, are excellent antioxidants, anti-inflammatory and anticancer.

Raspberry (rubus, idaeus)

It's the richest fiber (7.4 gr). Excellent source of vitamins, minerals, polyphenols and anthocyanins that are good antioxidants and anti-inflammatory. Chronic diseases of rheumatic origin can benefit quite a lot, such as digestion for the supply of soluble fibers. It contains ellagic acid which prevents damage to cellular DNA.

Blackberry (Rubus Fructicous).

They gather in the middle of summer in the woods. The presence of anthocyanins (dark color) confers an antioxidant and protective power of the ¿endothelium of arterial vessels. Excellent source of vitamins, minerals (Na, K, Ca, Fe, Ph). Good potassium content that is 260 mg , but is in first place among fruits and vegetables, as Iron content (1.6 gr).Wild strawberry (Fragaria/vesca)

Contains anthocyanins and ellagic acid, carcinogenicity inhibitors. Thanks to the presence of polyphenols they protect the cardiovascular system. They promote intestinal functions due to the presence of soluble fibers, are low-calorie, purifying, detoxifying, refreshing and help lower pressure.

Antioxidants

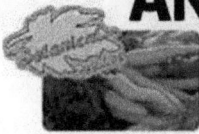

"Antioxidants are substances that can prevent or slow damage to cells caused by free radicals, unstable molecules that the body produces as a reaction to environmental and other pressures."

https://www.medicalnewstoday.com/articles/301506

ANTIOXIDANTS

Carrots — Betacarotene
Garlic — Allicin
Lemon — Hesperidin
Tomatoes — Licopene

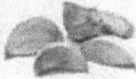

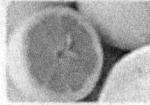

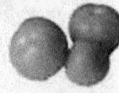

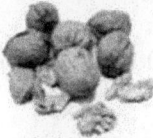

Walnuts — Tocopherols
Black grapes — Resveratrol
Broccoli — Glutathione
Apple — Quercetin

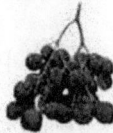

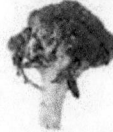

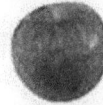

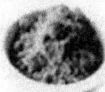

Turmeric — Curcumin
Onions — Quercetin
Green tea — Cathechin
Peppers — Capsanthin

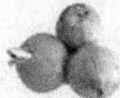

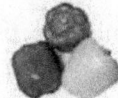

https://www.botanical-online.com/en/
medicinal-plants/antioxidants

TOP 10 ALKALINE FOODS

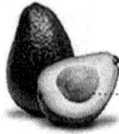 AVOCADO

SPINACH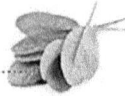

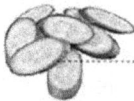 CUCUMBER

SEAWEED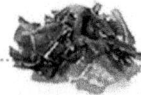

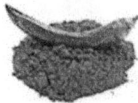 CAYENNE PEPPER

KALE

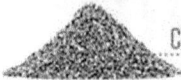 CHIA SEEDS

WATERMELON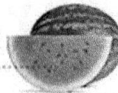

 LEMON

GARLIC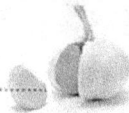

https://tangeetaughtu.com/2014/10/26/top-10-alkaline-foods/

Vegetables

All these foods never forget to be present in our daily menu. The beneficial properties of cabbage and the cruciferous family (cauliflower, cabbage, savoy cabbage, kale, red cabbage, kale, Brussels sprouts, broccoli, turnip tops, radish, arugula and horseradish.) are multiple. thanks to the large amount of mineral salts. Glucosinolates are important for antitumor properties. They are natural anti-Inflammatory (omega 3), anti-cancer, anti-oxidant, and anti-depressant.

Garlic/Onion/Leek

A nice family of nutrients that have substances in common with sulfur atoms. Allicin has anti-cancer properties, disinfectants, depurative, immunostimulant, vermifuge and excellent for controlling pressure and cholesterol.

CHAPTER 7

FIBERS

Talking about lifestyle and nutrition in the previous chapter, in particular, about vegetables, I realized that I have not highlighted enough the importance of fiber. I always recommend to all my patients to limit carbohydrates and eat more fiber, so let's see why.

The major benefits of a fiber-rich diet can be summarized as follows

i.   Normalizes bowel movements

ii.   Lowering cholesterol

iii.   Helps maintain bowel health

iv.   Aids in achieving healthy weight

v.   Helps control blood sugar levels. A high-fiber meal slows down the digestion of food into the intestines, which may help to keep blood sugars from rising rapidly.

vi.   Weight control: A high-fiber diet may help keep you fuller longer, which prevents overeating and hunger between meals.

vii.   Reduce the risk of type two diabetes and cardio vascular diseases.

viii. May prevent intestinal cancer: Insoluble fiber increases the bulk and speed of food moving through the intestinal tract, which reduces time for harmful substances to build up.

Constipation: Constipation can often be relieved by increasing the fiber or roughage in your diet. Fiber works to help regulate bowel movements by pulling water into the colon to produce softer, bulkier stools. This action helps to promote better regularity. Helps you live longer? Maybe yes.

But there is also another consideration, perhaps curious, perhaps bizarre, to highlight. It is believed that brain and intestine are in continuous contact, where there is a remarkable exchange of information but also emotions. Their link is so strong that the intestine is often considered as a second brain. Thus, it seems that keeping the gut clean is, as it were, cleaning up, or putting in order the mind and clearing the brain. But that's not all, there's something else...interesting!

Meanwhile, let's see what these fibers are and where they come from.

What is fiber?

Fiber is the structural part of plant foods – such as fruits, vegetables, and grains – that our bodies cannot digest or break down. It is split into two broad categories based on its water solubility. There are two kinds of fiber: soluble and insoluble.

Soluble fiber dissolves in water and can be metabolized by the 'good' bacteria in the dissolves in water to form a gummy gel. It can slow down the passage of food from the stomach to the intestine. Examples include dried beans, oats, barley, bananas, potatoes, and soft parts of apples and pears.

Insoluble fiber: often referred to as "roughage" because it does not dissolve in water. It holds onto water, which helps produce softer, bulkier stools to help regulate bowel movements. Examples include whole bran, whole grain products, nuts, corn, carrots, grapes, berries, and peels of apples and pears.

If we consider that the intestine is populated by an incredible number of bacteria (10 times more than all the cells in our body) that we can divide into two large families of good and bad bacteria that are constantly warring.

Fibers are the nourishment of good bacteria.

This is the most important reason that (some) dietary fibers are essential for health. They feed the "good" bacteria in the intestine, functioning as prebiotics. In this way, they promote the growth of "good" gut bacteria, which can have various positive effects on health.

How much fiber should I eat?

The Academy of Nutrition and Dietetics (USA) recommends consuming about 25-35 grams of total fiber per day, with 10-15 grams from soluble fiber or 14g of fiber per 1,000 calories. This can be accomplished by choosing 6 ounces of grains (3 or more ounces from whole grains), 2½ cups of vegetables, and 2 cups of fruit per day (based on a 2,000 calorie/day pattern). However, as we age, fiber requirements decrease. For those over the age of 70, the recommendation for women is 21 grams and for men 30 grams of total fiber per day.

CHAPTER 8

TIPS FOR BETTER FASTING

Advantages of fasting
....

Hunger and satiety
....

Intermittent fasting
....

Suggestions
....

An appropriate diet, as we have seen, can be of valuable help for health problems and good prevention. A frugal diet is always good, but even better would be...fasting. It seems trivial, but it seems to be the best medicine. Our organism, in the course of evolution, has adapted well to this situation and has learned to take advantage of it for our health. Today, beyond a sort of popular wisdom, it is also scientifically proven that fasting is a very useful way to stay fit and healthy.

We know that fasting is a form of behavior practiced in ancient times both out of necessity, when there was a lack of food, and as a choice dictated by religious beliefs, even by people of different histories and cultures.

A Japanese researcher was awarded the 2016 Nobel Prize in Medicine. His research demonstrated the very benefits of fasting. Dr. Yoshinor Ioshumi claims that during fasting, interesting transformations take place in our bodies that are incredibly healthy. In particular the autophagy, in other words, the fact of being able to feed on our waste and clean our body.

The main advantages are many and well known. It is a fact that those who can observe this behavior discover a certain sense of lightness and in the end feel much better. On a psychological level, the practice of fasting improves will-power and self-control and in the long run we get used to be less hungry and eat less and less. Some famous sages and scholars say that fasting also cleanses and purifies the mind. The battle against the primal instinct to eat can be hard, sometimes, but there are tricks that can help us to win. We'll look at some of them.

How the sense of hunger works.

The regulation of the sensation of hunger and satiety is quite complex and is based on the hypothalamus, that part of the brain that has the task of keeping under control some of the variables of our organism, such as sleep and wakefulness, hot and cold, stress and relaxation and also, precisely, hunger and satiety. The participants in this regulation are many. Hormones such as leptin, ghrelin, insulin, cortisol, serotonin, dopamine, norepinephrine, neuropeptide Y (NPY) and others with the vagus nerve.

However, simplifying, we can imagine a competition between these two hormones: leptin and ghrelin that try to convince the hypothalamus to make a decision.

Do I need to eat or not?

The sense of satiety is regulated by a hormone called Leptin (derived from leptos which in Greek means thin, slender) It has the task of sending the signal to the brain that we no longer need to eat. It is produced by fat cells and its receptors are located in the hypothalamus. (ventromedial area).

For example, when the stomach is full, leptin is activated, which together with the vagus nerve sends the signal to the brain that we no longer need to eat. Unfortunately, this signal is not instantaneous, that is, it arrives with a delay, so that we continue to eat even when we don't need it anymore. And so, eating slowly can be a good trick to wait for the signal of satiety and not to eat more than we have to.

Its antagonist, the hormone that induces appetite, is called ghrelin, produced mainly in the stomach, but also in the intestine and is activated when the stomach is empty. Or when we smell food or see food or even for a certain habit of being hungry at a certain time of day. There is another actor in this process that is cortisol, the stress hormone. Cortisol is a hormone produced by the adrenal glands. Its main action is to induce an increase in blood sugar. This results in an increased feeling of hunger.

Here's a little help to make it easier with....

Three suggestions.

Here is the first suggestion ... behavioral type

So when you fast it would be good practice to be as relaxed and quiet as possible to not activate the 'increase of cortisol, then welcome meditative practices, relaxing breathing (excellent diaphragmatic), yoga, music, etc. Occupy your mind in engaging activities, so that you have something to do to fill the waiting time before starting to eat again. Prepare a few days before with a healthy lifestyle by eliminating meat, alcohol, coffee and increasing consumption of fruits and vegetables, preferably, raw.

Second tip...start a little at a time

Today, intermittent fasting is very fashionable, it works very well, it is feasible without particular effort and at the same time it also allows you not to give up satisfying, sometimes and in moderation, that primal instinct to eat. You can easily get used to it as a lifestyle. You can start, for example, by trying to skip a meal (better not to skip breakfast). Many people suggest, perhaps even better, to eat only one meal, even if it is abundant.

Third suggestion......use auriculotherapy

I will talk about it at greater length in the next chapter, but in two lines I can anticipate that auriculotherapy or also called neuromodulation is a typical discipline of integrative medicine. This was discovered in France in the middle of last century and rediscovered only recently. It is based on the principle that on the surface of the auricle there is a representation or map of the structures and functions of the entire organism. There are particular points that are related to activities of the nervous system. There are, for example, points related to the stomach, mouth, pancreas, but also to stress, allergies and, incidentally, the stimulus of hunger.

How does Auriculotherapy work?

Stimulating certain points of the auricle activates mechanisms that rebalance certain functions of the body, such as neuromodulators, endorphins and hormones. With regard to hunger, there are interesting studies that hypothesize that the stimulation of certain points can reduce appetite by suppressing ghrelin, the hormone that antagonizes leptin. There is a particular protuberance, easily identifiable in the auricle, called trago, easy to treat, where the point of hunger resides. So if you can treat this point with a certain pressure with the index finger and thumb, that is squeezing between the two fingers you can get a certain stimulation. However, there is also a more complete and complex procedure of acupuncture, with the stimulation of precise points on the body and in the ear, for weight limitation/hunger control. You will find it in the appendix on 'weight control'.

CHAPTER 9

TIPS AND TRICKS FOR A BETTER QUALITY OF SLEEP.

This is a delicate and very interesting topic that deserves great attention, because it is of fundamental importance both for a correct and healthy lifestyle, and in general to maintain a state of health that is the basis for good prevention. It is thought, in fact, and modern scientific medicine confirms it, that a large majority of diseases, today, can be, in time, well preventable.

The subject is much more complex than it may seem and difficult to treat in a complete and thorough way.

I will limit myself to indicate some suggestions probably less known to the general public.

For a healthy lifestyle, in addition to diet and physical activity, we should also pay attention to how we recharge our body, mind and spirit. Rest is like the string of a bow that is stretched to shoot the arrow... if the string is stretched well with the right strength the arrow will run away with a certain energy, but if the rest is not of good quality, the bow will not be well stretched and the arrow will not go very far. Banal consideration, even more banal to underline that rest is important, however we do not always give it the right importance.

Disorders related to inadequate sleep or bad rest are quite frequent, but fortunately there are all kinds of remedies, natural and not, traditional and not. And last but not least, the grandmother's remedy: warm milk and honey in winter, chamomile tea and hot bath, essential oil of lavender and ginger that always works.

But let us go to the root of the problem and let us try to guess the easiest, most common and intuitable causes, in general, of those who suffer from this disorder, keeping in mind that each of us is different with own particular story. We can however assume that bad habits, both of food and behavior, particular situations where there is at the center a situation of little serenity or conflict or stress, are a group of causes to be taken into serious consideration.

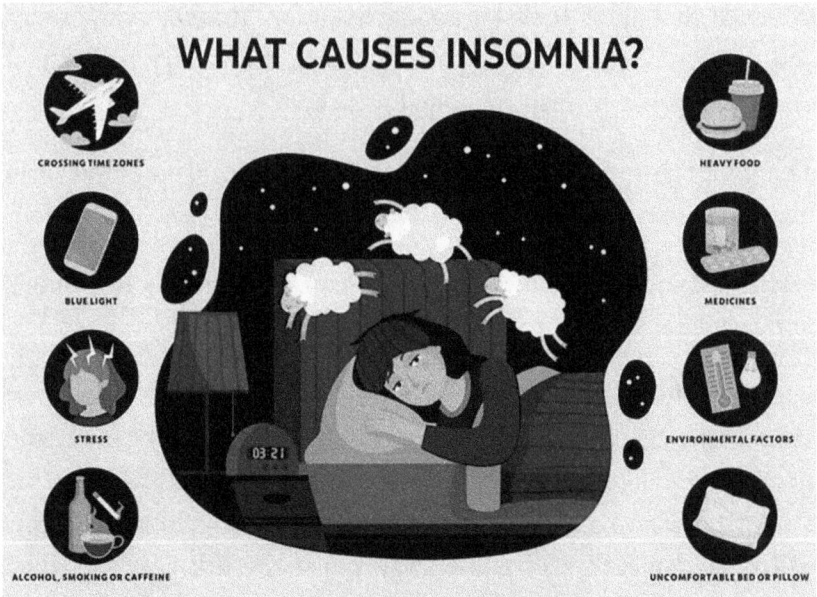

Importance of vitamin D

Often forgotten by all, but a good level of vitamin D is essential for good health. It has been repeatedly shown that a deficiency of this vitamin is often found in many diseases, including insomnia.

Vitamin D is a fat-soluble vitamin that plays a critical role in several aspects of health, related in a strict sense to the exposure to sunlight. It favors the absorption, at intestinal and renal level, of calcium, an essential mineral for a correct mineralization and for the maintenance of compactness and health of bones and teeth. It is estimated that, today, with the lack of exposure to the sun, the vast majority of the population is deficient in Vitamin D.

Before continuing, I would like to remind you of the definition of some of the players in this study....Cortisol, melatonin, magnesium, and other minerals involved.

Cortisol is a steroid hormone that your adrenal glands, the endocrine glands on top of your kidneys, produce and release. Cortisol affects several aspects of your body and mainly helps regulate your body's response to stress.

Melatonin.

Melatonin is a hormone naturally produced by the body that signals to the brain that it is time to go to sleep. Improving its level can help improve sleep quality.

Stress.

A key concept and fundamental around which revolves a set of mental activities, feelings, emotions and so on.

We can consider it under two aspects, one positive (eustress) and another negative (distress).

But where does this stress come from?

Under normal conditions, *eustress* is an excellent life-saver that in itself would not be a bad thing, that is, it is activated by the sympathetic autonomic nervous system that gives the drive to action. It gives us the charge to fight or flee in the face of imminent danger or puts us in a condition of active vigilance, lucidity and desire to do something positive and of great help to the action, but often, even when we do not need it anymore, it remains harnessed on us as discomfort and becomes a kind of continuous worry. And this is the kind of stress we have to fight, the *distress*. How to do it? Keep cortisol, the stress hormone, at bay.

Cortisol is produced by the adrenal glands, stimulated by signals it receives from the hypothalamus. It is activated in the morning and has its own circadian cycle. It slowly decreases from the afternoon onwards.

It is very sensitive to glycemia, that is to the level of sugar in the blood and is activated together with insulin. It should be kept low, especially in the evening, another reason to limit carbohydrates at dinner and/ or large meals.

Excessive physical activity in the evening should also be discouraged, because it creates stress and activates cortisol.

In addition to cortisol, the biological clock is also driven by another hormone, melatonin, called the hormone of well-being, of tranquility, which is opposed to it.

An important role to manage this balance could be the choice of a diet aimed to encourage a good level of melatonin and discourage the increase of cortisol.

Melatonin, the hormone of well-being, is produced by the epiphysis (or pineal gland), a gland located at the back of the brain, from tryptophan, an amino acid which is converted into serotonin, which in turn is transformed into melatonin.

The Third Eye

It is hypothesized that manual stimulation of the third eye can promote the production of melatonin, but also indirectly improve self-awareness, increase mental power and elevate spirituality

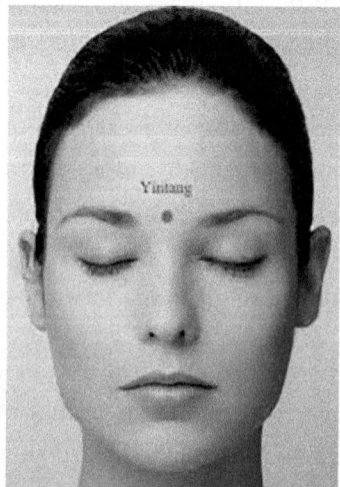

The third eye is located on the forehead in the center of the eyebrows. The Chinese call it Yin Tang (the room of seals) magical point that activates the 'intuition ... reduces the fog of the

brain and opens the mind. This point is considered the seat of the shen (spirit).

The pineal gland, or epiphysis, is an endocrine gland of the vertebrate brain, producing melatonin, which is responsible for sleep-wake balance and circadian rhythm. It is thought that the third eye and this gland are somehow in communication.

The pineal gland, known in ancient times both by Galen* as the *organ of sacredness*, and by Descartes**, who considered it *the seat of the soul.*

This gland also has another reflex point in the ear. As we will see in the study of auricular therapy, in the ear you can find many reflex points of the body.

This point is located at the base of the *intertragic incisura*, in an area easily accessible by the fingers and stimulation.

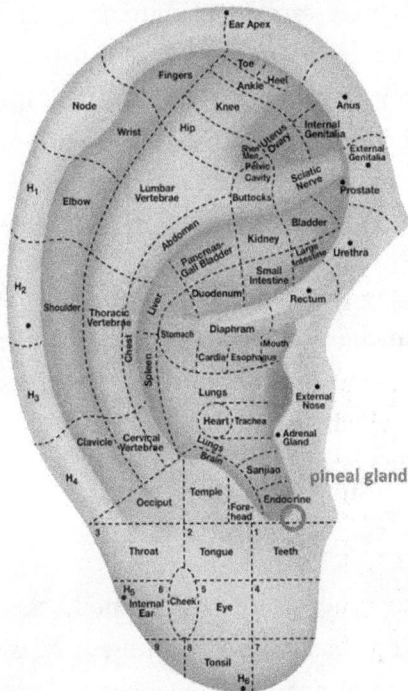

So manual stimulation of these two points (third eye and the pineal gland point on the ear) is of great help in encouraging the production of melatonin.

This can be of great use when our circadian cycle is disturbed and disrupted for some reason such as long plane rides at different longitudes (jet lag) or long night shifts.

Another small suggestion would be to steer our diet in this direction.

Fortunately there are several foods rich in melatonin:

- in fruits: apples, pomegranates, cherries, bananas
- in dried fruit: peanuts, almonds, walnuts and pistachios.
- in vegetables: onions cucumbers cabbage, asparagus
- adaptogenic herbs: ginseng, astragalus, licorice
- Ginger and cocoa are also good sources.

About cocoa it is necessary to pay attention to the quantity and percentage of sugar to which it is mixed to make chocolate. (the best would be the 90% bitter one) and to think it is also a source of caffeine, which obviously would not help sleep. Among other things, cocoa also contains a good quantity of magnesium (519 mg per 100 gr.). Magnesium is also a mineral which is connected with stress.

If one could manage to arrange nutrition and relaxation one would already be well on the way, however, integrative medicine has also made available classic protocols for both sleep disorders and those related to anxiety, which sometimes overlap.

We have already seen two simple examples of acupressure and auriculotherapy.

But there are also other points of the body that are sensitive to pressure and cause a certain state of pleasant relaxation. (The other points are described in detail in the appendix, where we treat both stress and insomnia. They are located on the face, hands, wrists, chest, feet and ankles and the auricle.)

Let us now look at two points on the foot and one above the ankle that have an ancient history of being very effective points for combating both insomnia and stress reduction. The first is an extra meridian point that is located in the center of the heel. Its name is Extra point Shimian M-LE-5.

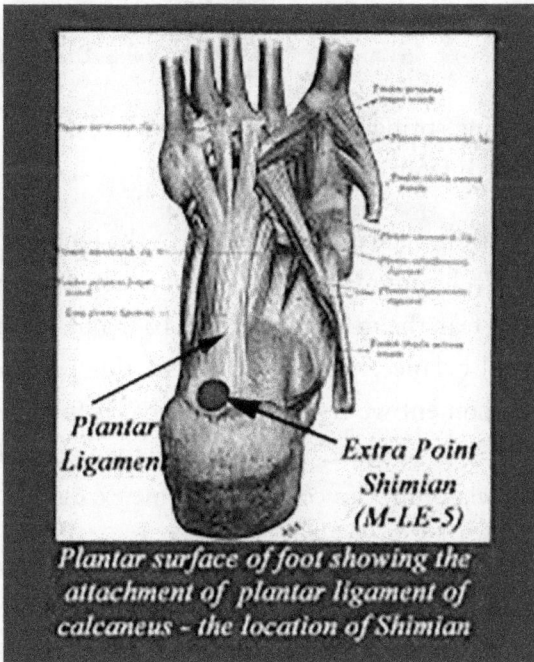

Plantar surface of foot showing the attachment of plantar ligament of calcaneus - the location of Shimian

The second is the first point of the K 1 kidney meridian which is located centrally at one third of the extremity, between the second and third metatarsal bones. A very famous point and often responsive to pressure. A point directly related to stress.

ACUPUNCTURE POINT OF THE WEEK

Kidney 1

Yongquan

Used to treat

- Headache
- Blurry vision
- Dizziness
- Sore throat
- Dry tongue
- Loss of voice
- Loss of conciousness

#TipTuesday

AOMA

Spirit of the Acupuncture Points

Kidney 1

BUBBLING SPRING

Spiritual Level Indications:

- Brings a surge of revitalizing, restoring & invigorating energy
- Restores hope & optimism when feeling utterly depleted

P.S. You are invited! Join our online community and engage with your holistically inspired peers
Community.VillageWellness.net

The name, gushing spring, makes good the idea of energy and vitality that takes strength from the earth.

The Kidney Meridian starts from the sole of the foot and reaches the collarbone (K 27, elegant mansion) and is connected to water and this to the feeling of fear, the mother of stress. To maintain, or restore, an adequate mental balance, the stimulation of this point can be very useful. If for a moment we try to imagine that mental agitation and stress (cortisol) are associated with the fire, then the water (kidney meridian and melatonin) can counteract some excess.

Chinese medicine says that the kidneys belong to water and the heart to fire: therefore it is believed that Kidneys and Heart help each other. The harmony between kidneys and heart is one of the prerequisites for a stable and tranquil *shen*.

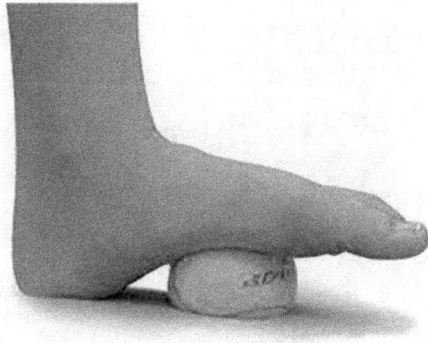

this can be another way to stimulate K1

Who is this mysterious shen?

Shen is a difficult term to define and translate, it is a concept that lies at the center of our mind. The mind, the spirit, the soul, the psyche...a very subtle energy that guides our thoughts and regulates our emotions. Shen is based in the heart. As all emotions are based in the heart. The primary goal of maintaining health is to calm the Shen, should it be in agitation or simply upset.

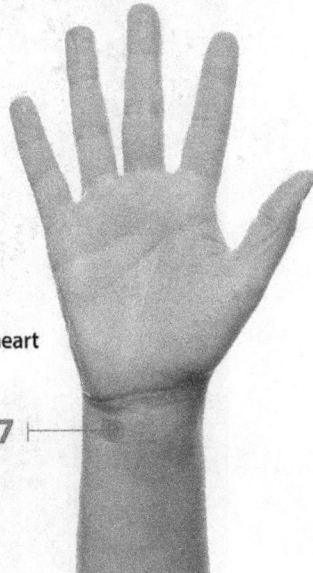

MODERN REFLEXOLOGY

HT 7

- Helps calm the mind
- Nourishes heart blood and helps with insomnia anxiety
- It can be used to strengthen the heart

HT 7

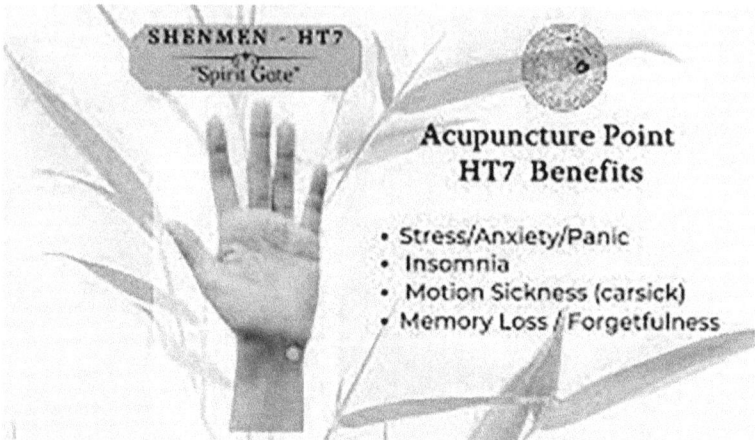

SHENMEN - HT7
"Spirit Gate"

Acupuncture Point HT7 Benefits

- Stress/Anxiety/Panic
- Insomnia
- Motion Sickness (carsick)
- Memory Loss / Forgetfulness

A curious thing that I wanted to point out is that the two most important points that work on relaxation, which are located on the wrist and the other in the ear have the same name: the SHEN MEN. Which could be translated, simply, as the door of the spirit, or heavenly door.

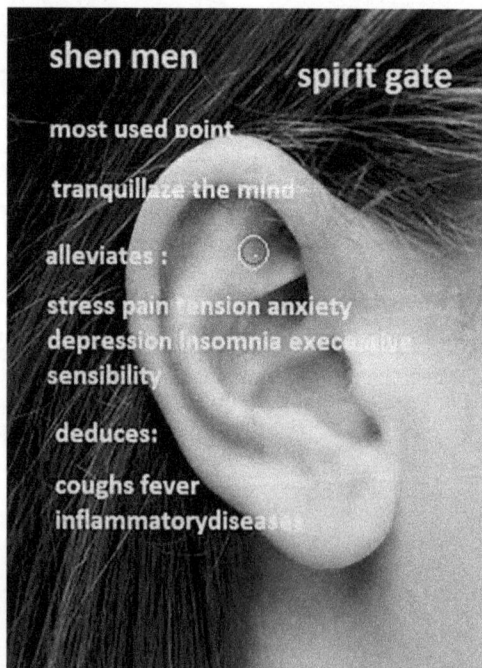

shen men   spirit gate

most used point

tranquillaze the mind

alleviates :

stress pain tension anxiety
depression insomnia execcutive
sensibility

deduces:

coughs fever
inflammatorydiseases

Shen has its natural seat in the heart. When it is positive it becomes happiness, love, passion, when it is negative it brings bad thoughts and worries. So the term **Shen Men** could be associated with a door, which once opened or unlocked, lets out all the negativity, freeing and purifying the mind.In the ear is located at the top of the triangular dimple.

In my opinion, a technique that works very well is deep breathing combined with Yoga or other relaxation techniques (autogenic training). Also singing in a choir, reciting mantras, listening to good music (Gregorian chants) can be of great help to relieve stress and to sleep better.

I forgot to tell you that laughing has been discovered in recent studies (see the yoga of laughter) to be a good tranquilizer, as well as devoting.

There can still be many suggestions to improve the quality of sleep. We will see some other points that can help if stimulated regularly,

Let us contend to remember these 6 points:

Yintang – third eye
ht 7 shenmen on the wrist
shen men and pineal gland on the ear
shimian and K 1 on the foot

CAUSES OF DISEASES....
HUMIDITY

Origin

Difficult to make classifications about the causes of diseases today, it would be too complicated, but the ancient doctors had simply grouped them into three different factors:

1   **Of internal origin:** emotions, stress, anger, sadness, fear, brooding, etc.
2   **Of external origin:** climatic factors, heat, cold, wind, humidity, dryness

3   **Neither internal nor external origin:** lifestyle, diet, sleep, sexual life, psychophysical activity.

Humidity is one of the most important causes of disease; but often, it is hidden and ignored. It is a bit special because it can be considered both as an internal cause and, thinking of climatic factors, also an external cause.

Disorders Associated with Humidity

Humidity could be associated with numerous disorders such as:

- ➲ from **metabolic disorders** (diabetes 2, high cholesterol, obesity)
- ➲ from **states of inflammation** (arthritis, arthrosis, muscle pain, headaches)
- ➲ **allergies**, chronic fatigue, depression, drowsiness and sleep disorders, digestive difficulties and many others.

According to Chinese medicine, moisture is associated with the earth element and as the main organ with the spleen-pancreas.

Possible causes include:

Nutrition/diet

The Chinese historically do not like milk and dairy products. Have you ever seen a Chinese person eating cheese? You may have noticed that it is almost impossible to order cheese in a Chinese restaurant. However, it is also not recommended to eat starchy foods, sugars, cold foods (everything that is white is cold and leads to humidity), industrial foods, alcoholic beverages, even fruit should be consumed with a certain moderation.

Spicy, warming (ginger) and refreshing (bitters) foods are better.

FOODS THAT FORM DAMPNESS

- Sugar
- Yeast
- Wheat
- Saturated fats
- Roasted Peanuts
- Dairy products
- Bread
- Pork
- Bananas
- Concentrated juices

SP6

ST36

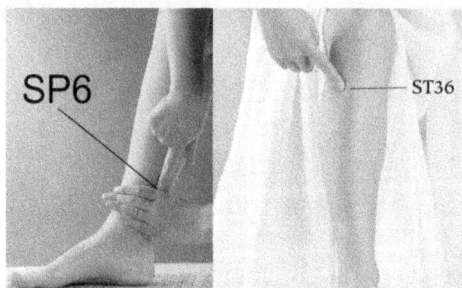

Sedentariness

Lack of physical activity, often linked to obesity, is certainly one of the possible causes; along with a poor lifestyle (poor sleep quality)

Stress and anxiety

Worries, sadness and depression slow down the activity of the organs responsible for the transformation and transport of fluids. Think of the pancreas (spleen) which is the organ dedicated to remorse. Repressed anger and resentment. Excessive intellectual effort, obsessive thinking.

Humid environments

Excess moisture in the environment where you live can cause mold and can provide an ideal habitat for bacteria and viruses.

Possible remedies may include the following:

Lifestyle

A set of attentions regarding diet, physical activity, stress reduction, good quality of sleep that are always at the base of all integrative therapies. Easy to say, but in fact if it were possible, it would have significant advantages on the final result. Often this alone would be enough to solve the majority of problems. There are foods that can invigorate the spleen and transform the dampness: spicy foods and those of a warm or lukewarm nature: cinnamon, pepper, shallots, leeks, ginger, soy, tofu.

Acupressure

According to Chinese medicine there are particular points on our body, scattered along the 12 energy meridians that are particularly sensitive to stimulation.

This stimulation can be done in various ways: with finger pressure (shiatzu, tuinà), with the insertion of thin needles (acupuncture), with the help of metal balls (magnetic) or seeds to stick near the points and with electrical stimulation. The effect does not change much. There are many points that can be taken into consideration according to different situations and causes. I would like to highlight one very special point, not only to solve the problem of humidity but also of many other disorders.

Massage this point everyday and THIS will happen to your body!

San Yin Jao SP 6

San Yin Jao SP 6

The inside of both feet

This is a very special point. It deserves special attention. Its name means intersection of the three yin meridians of the foot, namely spleen, kidney and liver.

So because of its position it influences all three of these meridians, thus toning the spleen and pancreas, stimulating liver function, toning the kidneys, and stimulating and promoting fluid circulation. Hence, the suggestive nickname of Master of Liquids – where there is a problem of liquids there must be the involvement of this point. Reflecting for a moment, it occurred to me that when I was studying the history of Western Medicine, it was fashionable to think that the origin of all diseases stemmed from a bad balance of our fluids, the famous four humors of Empedocles and Hippocrates.

History Memories

At the time of Hippocrates (460-357 BC), the fashionable theory was Empedocles, that is, it was thought that the concept of health and disease was based on the harmony and balance of the four humors (liquids): *blood, yellow bile, black bile, and phlegm.* It is no coincidence that the term humor derives from this. [from lat. humor or umor..humid].

The importance of *SP 6* lies in the fact that it is involved in a myriad of therapeutic solutions such as:

Irregular menstruation, dysmenorrhea, metrorrhagia, leucorrhea, amenorrhea, postpartum weakness, persistent lochia, infertility, nocturnal emission, spermatorrhea, impotence, premature ejaculation, penile pain, hernia, testicular atrophy, Enuresis, anuria, edema, dysuria Spleen and Stomach Deficiency, borborygmus, abdominal distension, diarrhea, foot paralysis, beriberi, muscle aches, skin diseases, hives, different types of Insomnia and not least resolves the moisture. (Not to be used during pregnancy.)

In addition to the famous *SP 6* point, there are 5 other points on our body that are particularly sensitive to treatment. Whether by massage or puncture or heat with moxibustion (1)

Ren 9 just above the navel, on the Ren Mai (conception vessel)

St 40 in the center of the leg on the stomach meridian

Sp 3 located on the foot on the spleen meridian

Sp 9 located in the knee area on the same meridian

Ki 7 located in the ankle area on the kidney meridian

Acupoints for getting rid of

DAMPNESS

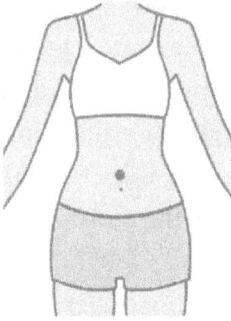 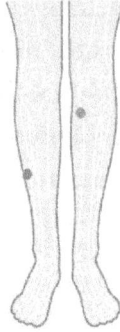 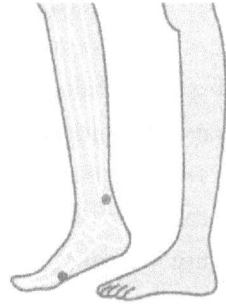

REN 9

Called "Shui Fen" meaning Water Separation can open up water passage and get rid of excess water.

Use moxa stick or moxa with ginger.

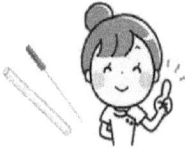

ST 40

Called " Feng Long" meaning Abundant Bulge is known as the Phlegm point.

SP 9

Called "Yin Ling Quan" meaning Yin Mound Spring drains dampness generally through urination.

SP 3

Called "Tai Bai" meaning Supreme White is the Yuan source point of the Spleen. It's where the Qi pools.

KI 7

Called "Fu Liu" meaning Recover Flow. Tonify Kidney Yang to regulate water metabolism. Good for sweating issues too.

WWW.KANPOBLISS.COM

Fenglong (ST-40)

◆ **Location**
At the midpoint of the line joining ST-35 and ST-41 and 2 fingerbreadths lateral to the anterior crest of the tibia or 1 fingerbreadth lateral to ST-38, between the extensor digitorum longus and peroneus brevis muscles.

◆ **Needling**
Vertically or obliquely 1–1.5 cun

◆ **Actions/Indications**
--- Transforms Dampness and Phlegm, clears Phlegm in the Lung and Heart, calms the shen

◆ **Special features**
Luo-connecting point. Main acupuncture point for eliminating Phlegm.

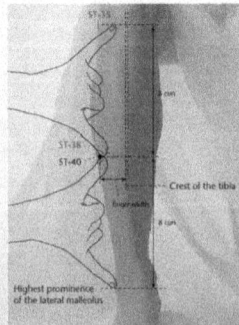

https://acumeridianpoints.com/stomach-st-40-fenglong/

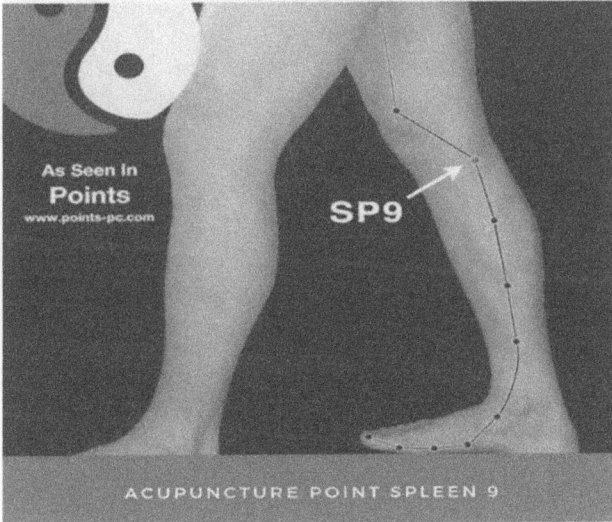

TRADITIONAL CHINESE MEDICINE

RESOLVING "DAMPNESS"

As Seen In
Points
www.points-pc.com

SP9

ACUPUNCTURE POINT SPLEEN 9

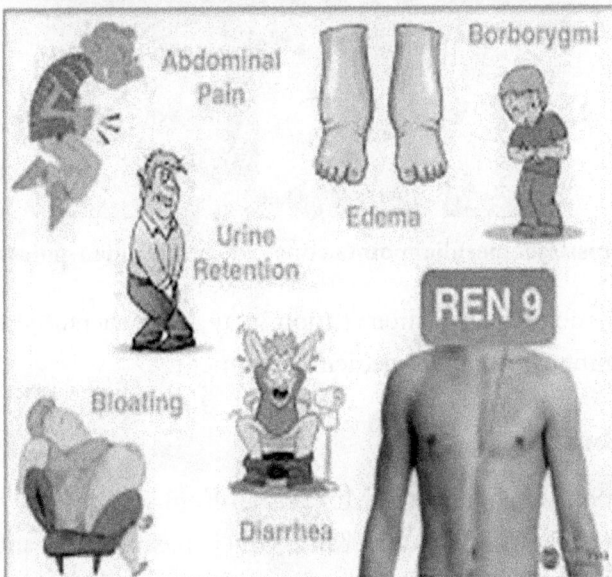

Abdominal Pain

Borborygmi

Urine Retention

Edema

REN 9

Bloating

Diarrhea

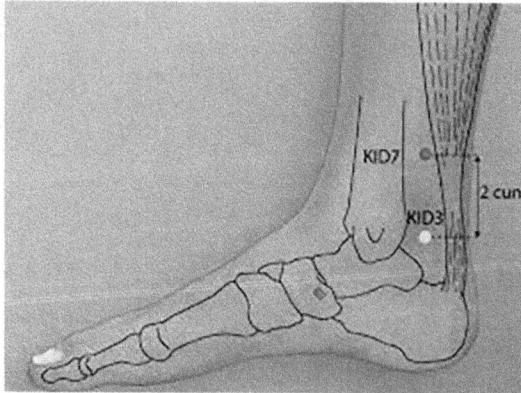

https://acumeridianpoints.com/kidney-meridian-points/

Other possibilities for intervention may be auriculotherapy and spleen toning with herbal medicine treatment.

(1) Moxibustion

Moxibustion (or abbreviated Moxa) is an English term derived from the Japanese words Moe and Kusa, which mean "burn" and "grass" (therefore "burning grass") and refer to the practice of a therapeutic technique that uses the heat developed by burning an herb (artemisia vulgaris) in correspondence of acupuncture points.

The ancient origin is found in documents dating back to the II-I century BC.

CHAPTER 11

THE LONG ROAD TO LONGEVITY

D elaying aging or to age in good health, is a very intriguing goal. Unfortunately, it requires a certain commitment and is not at all easy, giving up, sometimes, many pleasant things in life. According to some experts and scholars in the field, three main lines have been identified that can be followed. The first is a careful and healthy diet (life-style). The second is a constant physical activity. The third way is the one that involves that brain and mind. We have already highlighted the importance of proper nutrition, but I would still like to suggest a few more concepts.

Why Vegetarian?

I am not strictly vegetarian, I would like to be, (maybe one day I will be able to) because this behavior is appreciable both on an ethical level and also from the health point of view.

The scholars who have worked in this area of research are many, I would like to mention two in particular: Franco Berrino and T. Colin Campbell.

Dr. Franco Berrino, worked at the National Institute of Tumors in Milan, where he directed the Department of Preventive and Predictive Medicine. On the web, he has published numerous videos on his research on proper nutrition and lifestyle.

I quote some of his suggestions and teachings:

> Vegetarians are healthier and live longer.

> Meat eaters have a much higher
> risk of developing cancer.

> Physical activity and exposure to the
> sun are essential for good health.

> Frugality and fasting are, however,
> the best eating behaviors.

> We free the mind by singing,
> meditating, breathing.

The China Study (T. Colin Campbell) is a famous epidemiological study, lasting 27 years, on the relationship between diet and disease, carried out in collaboration with various universities, concludes, among other things, that:

Several types of cancer are related to excessive consumption of animal protein. The consumption of dairy products may increase the risk of prostate cancer.

Antioxidants present in fruits and vegetables are linked to better intellectual performance in old age.

Why Breakfast?

Most nutrition experts emphasize the importance of this meal. There is a popular saying that goes: eat breakfast like a king, lunch like a prince and dinner like a beggar. Not everyone agrees, but I join the majority. I like that theory (of the saving gene) of the primitive man, hunter-gatherer. Even today, we are the grandchildren (for about 24,000 generations) of the man who alternated fasting, hunger and abundance depending on the situations that were often unpredictable. Our direct ancestors had to get used, and adapt during the evolutionary path both to famine and to eat in quantity when they could, never having the certainty of what could happen in the following days. So it has developed in our DNA (still similar to 99% of that of the monkeys) a gene called "sparing" that should act like this. If in the morning there is food, it means that we are not in a famine and you can eat as much as you want, even without exaggerating because our body has the feeling of being calm – probably, there will be food during the day. If instead we don't eat in the morning, our organism supposes that we could be in a situation of famine. Therefore, it triggers the alarm and we tend to put aside what we will eat as soon as possible. From a research, in fact, it would result that the majority of those who skip breakfast have an abdominal circumference greater than the average allowed that is 95 cm for men and 80 cm for women. One way to keep this measure under control, trivially, is caloric restriction, physical activity and intermittent fasting.

Other researchers (such as Dr. Eugenio Origa, nutritionist, another teacher of the master of Integrative Medicine) argue that the absorption of nutrients introduced in the morning would be 30%, that of lunch 50% and 100% of the evening meal. In Chinese medicine it is thought that the stomach in the morning has the maximum energy and in the evening reaches its minimum. Therefore, it would be healthier to eat a lot in the morning than in the evening. There are also other hormonal considerations. Cortisol in the evening should be kept low in order not to counteract the serotonin that facilitates rest, recharge and sleep. This cortisol hormone, called stress hormone, is easily raised by insulin if you have a large dinner, or with carbohydrates.

What not to eat or, at least, limit:

Bad Eating Habits

By tradition and culture, sitting at the table is a pleasant magical moment of pleasure, sharing and relaxation and thinking about limitations is often really sad. With a little attention and some small sacrifice it is possible to find a balanced solution. It should be remembered that "we eat to live and not live to eat".

Dr. Carlo Maggio, a well-known cardiologist, during the course of Antiaging held at the University of Florence, cautioned that one should be careful with the four famous white poisons, so harmful, that make us age prematurely. Sugar is in first place, followed by salt, white flour, and milk and its derivatives.

Margarine is also white. Once it was thought to be a better product than butter, lighter and of vegetable origin. Today we have realized that it is not true. There are hydrogenated fats, additives and derivatives of palm oil, which many say is not too healthy.

Alcohol

Excessive consumption of wine, spirits, hard liquor. Varieties of alcohol, in general, are aggravating factors and can cause dehydration and acidification. Beer attracts prolactin which disturbs the hormonal balance. The liver, which is the organ most involved, can be seriously affected. Wine, which contains resveratrol, although an excellent antioxidant, should be consumed with great moderation.

Salt

The excessive consumption of salt and spicy foods, (except for ginger and turmeric) can also cause irritation. It is often found hidden. But where? In all preserved and baked products. But, not only that, it is found in all preserved products, salt being, since ever, an excellent preservative.

The damages could be many: high blood pressure, immune system, cardiovascular diseases, stroke and many others. Better to use gomasio (roasted sesame seeds) or soy sauce, or iodized salt. The American Heart Association (AHA) suggests that most adults should reduce their intake to just 1,500 milligrams per day, of salt, in order to maintain low blood pressure levels.

A good idea, suggested by many, is to drink plenty of water. Good hydration dilutes salts, possibly in excess and, also brings a good sense of satiety.

It is usual to say that one needs to drink about 2 liters of water per day, with possible differences depending on changes of season, psychophysical situation, heat or medication intake.

To determine the exact amount, you should drink based on your body weight, you can follow the following calculation: 30 ml x kg body weight = ml per day.

Red Meats

Abuse of meat, especially red meat, animal fats, sausages, processed or refined foods that lead to acidosis or increased uric acid. Some claim that red meat is carcinogenic. Many suggest limiting their use. In general, vegetarians are healthier and have fewer problems, but they should supplement their diet with Vitamin B12.

Red meat also has another problem. The processing, their preservation and the way they are cooked often modify the molecules present which can become harmful. Foods of animal origin contain, besides proteins, many other substances such as saturated fats and iron in the heme group. In excessive doses, they can cause an increase in cholesterol, insulin levels in the blood and inflammation of the intestinal tract, increasing the risk of certain diseases, including cancers, in particular colorectal ones.

Milk and Dairy Products

Milk and dairy products should also be avoided or at least limited for several reasons. They contain, in fact, growth hormones (GF-1, GH) that favor the further development of prostate cells. Unfortunately, the milk that is produced (hormones and preservatives), today is not a food to be recommended. Cheeses can be one of the causes of humidity and of the many problems that derive from it. I have devoted an entire chapter.

Carbohydrates

This is a much-debated topic. There are those who argue that sugars are the main culprits of many diseases and disorders. Unfortunately, in the much vaunted, Mediterranean diet, carbohydrates are present in a percentage higher than 50%. In modern nutritional theories and in particular in the anti-aging ones, it is believed that carbohydrates should be drastically reduced in favor of fiber.

Our intestines are home to billions and billions of bacteria, viruses, fungi and other microbes that can be divided into two large families: the good and the bad. Ideally, there should be a certain balance between the two.

The first ones love fibers and the second ones love carbohydrates.

Nancy Appleton, a famous American nutritionist from the University of California, in her book Killer Sugar lists, comments and justifies as many as 140 ways in which sugar damages our health. To simplify, here are just a few. Obesity, diabetes, increases cholesterol and triglycerides, dysbiosis, tumors, cardiovascular problems, etc.

To complete the picture of suggestions for longevity, we are still missing the road of movement and meditation.

I do not want to talk about the benefits of the good habit of exercising regularly, because it has become almost trivial, everyone knows it. More difficult to tell and suggest is how to clean the mind, with meditation and other methods.

There are two paths to take. One is that of cleansing, i.e., freeing the mind from stress and other wastes that cloud free thinking and bring back lucidity. Another is to keep the brain active, training it to work, as if it were a muscle, continuously stimulating it to do its job, to imagine, to solve questions, to study, to write.

Develop a certain creativity by fantasizing about the future.

Conclusions

In summary, my recipe for delaying aging, and according to the latest research, could be:

Eat little, keep slim, occasionally fast;

Eat quality foods possibly not processed, fresh and local;

Prefer a vegetarian diet;

Avoid red meat, saturated fat;

Minimize carbohydrates, salt, dairy products;

Abound in fruits and vegetables;

Drink a lot of water;

Constantly exercise;

Keep your mind clean with meditation, breathing;

Listen and enjoy music, sing, dance and laugh;

Keep the brain alive with mental exercises,
always feed new interests;

Living in harmony with the environment,
enjoying the affections of friends, family, helping others;

See the next Chapter about the centenarians;

It is believed that the genetic factor influences
longevity by 10-20%, but that genes can be changed by nutrition.

CHAPTER 12

IN SEARCH OF THE BEST DIET

Centenarians

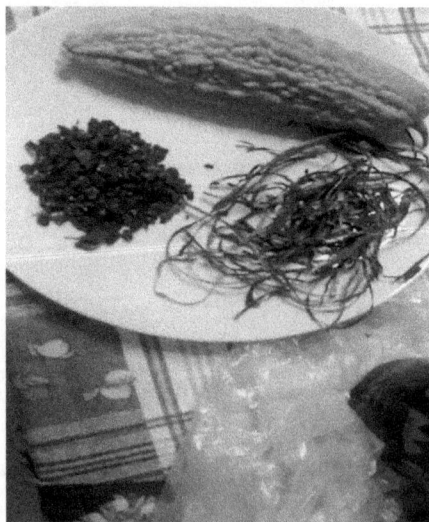

The secret to the longevity of the Japanese is probably hidden within these somewhat unusual foods: green tea, seaweed and this strange cucumber with a very bitter taste.

The Best Diet

For years, nutritionists and researchers in the field are still looking for it and are already thinking about giving up. Simply because such an ideal universal diet does not exist. The guidelines, in general, address everyone, and therefore no one, in particular, because we are all different, by age, physical and mental conditions, genetic predispositions, etc. and what might be good for you, is sometimes harmful to me. (However, there are some general recommendations, dictated by common sense, which is always good to keep in mind) It is not the food itself that we are looking for but the solution to delay aging or even better to age without getting sick. It is therefore not the food we eat that could be the root problem, but what we do not eat.

The curious story about centenarians.

From recent statistics have been identified some regions of the globe where many centenarians live or where the average life span is very high.

These small areas scattered in various parts of the world at different latitudes are called blue-zones and are, at the moment, five

From Wikipedia, the free encyclopedia.

'Blue Zone is a term used to identify a demographic and/or geographic area of the world in which life expectancy is significantly higher than the world average. The concept was born when scholars Gianni Pes and Michel Poulain published in Experimental Gerontology their demographic study on human longevity, which identifies the province of Nuoro, Sardinia, as the area with the highest concentration of centenarians in the world. Dan Buettner identified the island of Okinawa (Japan); Sardinia (Italy); Nicoya (Costa Rica); Icaria (Greece); and the Adventist community of Loma Linda, California, as hubs of longevity in the world, offering empirical data and firsthand observations in support.'

Some researchers, nutritionists, journalists and other curious people went to see how things really worked in those areas to check and possibly identify some of the secrets of their good health. Let's see what they discovered.

Sardinia (Nuoro)

In Sardinia, there are isolated villages where people still live as they did many years ago.

These simple people, who live in mostly mountainous and isolated areas, ate everything, even those foods that would be condemned by our classic nutritionists, such as milk, cheese, pasta, meat and wine. (Cannonau, very strong in revestrarol, good antioxidant)

They ate, that is, everything and only what was around their environment, fresh and natural foods. The cuisine, very simple although varied, follows the ancient recipes of the grandmother. The methods of cooking and processing of food is simple and traditional. In the surroundings there are no supermarkets, they even do not eat fish, even though they live on an island, because it is not available nearby. In these areas you can breathe an air of peaceful harmony, tranquility and where great is felt the warmth and affection of the family. It seems that there is no such thing as the feeling of our times, what we call stress.

So the secret of their good health lies in the fact that they do not eat foods that are preserved, processed and otherwise treated by the modern food industry. All those poisons that we ingest without even knowing it, in large quantities in almost all the food we find at the market.

The secret is all here: natural foods, directly from the earth, fresh and locally available, cooked at home in the traditional way, without any additives and in a peaceful and stress-free environment, with lots of outdoor physical activity.

This is a common denominator found in all of these regions, but with some differences related to their culture.

Okinawa

Japan is in itself one of the countries with longer-life-span of its citizens. Their meal is enriched with a very healthy cuisine: fish, soy, miso, seaweed, green tea, but in the island of Okinawa, which has remained a bit isolated, there is a greater number of centenarians than in the rest of the country.

Okinawans generally consume about 1,200 calories a day, far fewer than the 2,000 calories consumed by mainland Japanese.

They follow, in fact, the principles of "Hara Hachi Bun", (which means 80% stomach) a Confucian philosophy that recommends eating only until you are 80% full and chewing slowly. Seaweeds are used a lot, in particular nori, kombu and hijiki. Very present on the table are also legumes, mainly represented by soy. From the menu of this style of alimentation are, instead, practically absent or rarely consumed dairy products.

On the table of Okinawans is sometimes found a fruit known as Bitter Melon, which is not very common in the rest of the country, resembling a cucumber with a small sized knurled skin and an extremely bitter taste. It seems that this food possesses some incredible properties.

Momordica Charantia, also called bitter lemon, has inside an innumerable quantity of active principles and nutrients. Inside we can find:

Vitamins A, B, C, folic acid, mineral salts (iron, calcium, potassium, zinc, phosphorus), fibers, flavonoids (lutenin, zeaxanthin and quercetin), and saponins.

Perhaps quercetin is the secret of their longevity? (*)

But there is a strange exception that they sometimes eat, contrary to the general sense of health, which is pork. Probably they use it occasionally and certainly in limited quantities.

Loma Linda

For example, in California, there is a village where the Loma Linda Adventist community lives. Here everybody is very religious, wine is forbidden and the diet must be strictly vegetarian.

Ikaria island

On the island of Ikaria, in the Aegean Sea, you can eat anything, as long as it is produced within the island. Wine, produced locally and without any additive, is also consumed with a certain freedom.

To recapitulate, if it were possible to point out a common line which unites these populations, some determining factors must be considered:

Simple and traditional eating behavior. Fresh foods, possibly locally grown, home cooked, mostly of vegetable origin, such as legumes and vegetables. Refusal of red and processed meats. Try to eat in moderation.

Regular free and outdoor physical activity.

A social structure that favors intense human relationships and puts the family, sometimes religion, at the center. A life, in harmony with nature, lived close to friends and without stress.

(*) The wonders of quercetin.

Quercetin is the flavonoid most commonly used for metabolic and inflammatory disorders and the main activity attributed to it is the antioxidant one. In fact, it helps to reduce the formation of free radicals and pro-inflammatory substances.

Are rich in quercetin berries, apples, onions, celery, cruciferous vegetables (cauliflower, broccoli) and radicchio, but the food that contains the highest amount of this precious antioxidant is the caper.

A very special centenarian: my father.

He was blessed with good health and lived to be 107 years old. He was a pharmacist for more than 50 years, (but never took any medicine) stopped working at 77. He had 5 children and a very quiet life, even though he went through the two world wars. The secret of his longevity remains a mystery, but some indication may come from the fact that he never smoked, drank and overindulged. He went to bed very early, and in the morning before breakfast he had already read the newspaper. I think the warmth and affection of his loved ones played a major role in prolonging the last years of his life.

CHAPTER 13

MCT AND LONGEVITY

Stomach 36

Neiguan Pc 6

Ganoderma lucidum

Goji berries

Chinese Medicine, rich in ancient traditions, could also provide us with some curious and interesting pointers. Specifically through the stimulation of two points:

Stomach 36 and Neiguan Pc 6

In Stomach 36 is probably the most famous point, the richest in stories and anecdotes, the most used in various combinations also called in ancient times the point of 100 diseases. About 1500 years ago Qin Cheng zu, imperial physician of the Song dynasty, said that this point cures all chronic diseases characterized by weakness of the stomach, spleen, kidneys and other organs and so on, I'm not going to make the list, which would be very long.

Longevity with Stomach 36

A nice story that I read, years ago, told of the magical effect on health and in particular on the longevity of people regularly used to do moxibustion on that point. (Moxibustion is an alternative to massage and acupuncture, it allows stimulation of points through heat)

From... http://longevitylifestyleplan.blogspot.com/2015/03/st36.html

"A Japanese folk tale from the Edo era (1603-1867) about farmer Manpei tells that when Manpei was asked whether he had any secret to maintaining long life, he answered that he had no secret other than burning moxa on acupoint Stomach 36 every day, just as his ancestors had done. It is recorded that Manpei lived 243 years, his wife, Taku, lived 242 and their son, Mankichi, lived 196 years.

In recent records, it is well known that Doctor Shimetaro Hara used to burn Moxa on his St-36 every day and he lived to be over 100 years of age

Scientific studies cited by Dr. Shui Yin Lo in his book, The Biophysics for Acupuncture and Health; found that normal subjects who received acupuncture on acupoint Stomach 36, increased telomerase levels.

Clinical research now posits that stimulating St-36 increases Maximum Oxygen Uptake. It is known that increased Maximum Oxygen Uptake prevents and improves recovery time from diseases such as hypertension and diabetes. Maximum Oxygen Uptake also decreases the cancer rate. Thus, we may assume that the modern idea of maintaining health by increasing Maximum Oxygen Uptake is based on the same mechanism as our traditional wisdom for attaining longevity by stimulating St 36.

St-36 is located on the network called the Stomach Meridian. Stimulation of St-36 not only enlivens the point but also the entire meridian and stomach organ. According to this classic medical theory, the organ and meridian of the stomach are a part of the foundation of our life energy. Thus, stimulation on St-36 not only affects the leg where St-36 is located, but also affects the health of the whole body."

Its name Zu San Li, means 3 distances on the leg (zu means leg, san means three and Li distance) It would derive from its position at the root of the tibialis anterior muscle which is located three distances (three cun) from the beginning of the leg. Others argue that the name comes from another story. The distance (LI) would be associated with the idea of a mile as a measure of distance. It is said, in fact, that Chinese soldiers on the march had the habit of stopping every three miles to rest and especially to massage this point to invigorate their tired.

Another interesting point to delay aging and prevent or limit the damage of those diseases very common in the elderly is the point 6 of the meridian of the Heart Master which is located in the inner part of the wrist.

Neiguan (PC 6), a classical and experimental acupuncture point, has been recorded in ancient Chinese medical literature for thousands years and is preferred effectively in treating cardiovascular disorders.

Since cardiovascular disorders are very frequent in the elderly and are still the first cause of death, it could be interesting to act, even on this point, among other easy to locate, with the continuous and regular stimulation of this point.

However, Chinese Medicine, in addition to acupuncture and acupressure, offers other suggestions to this problem, derived from numerous studies both current and from ancient traditions and experiments.

Medicinal plants and immortal foods.

Ganoderma lucidum
Goji berries

Historically, Taoist Monks had the record for longevity, often living beyond a hundred years without manifesting the common symptoms of aging.

A particular combination of medicinal plants played an important role in their exceptional longevity and the maintenance of their strength: they were called the "immortal foods" and, in the secret formulas for longevity.

Starting from the belief that there are no miraculous plants, but that the popular tradition has often emphasized some mushrooms, such as reishi, to which was then assigned the name of the mushroom of immortality

The reishi mushroom, also known as Ganoderma lucidum and lingzhi, is a fungus that grows in various hot and humid locations in Asia.

Within the mushroom, there are several molecules, including triterpenoids, polysaccharides and peptidoglycans, that may be responsible for its health effects.

Goji berries have been used in China for more than 2000 years.

Mentioned in the ancient herbalist manual Shennong Ben Cao Jing.

They are small, dried red berries and have a pleasant taste. They have an ancient tradition for healthy properties: they fight fatigue, and anxiety. Not surprisingly, they have an excellent level of antioxidant power.

According to an ancient legend, there was a well near a Tibetan temple around which grew many goji bushes. Many of the berries ended up in the water of the well, where pilgrims used to drink. With the passing of the years they noticed that those who drank the water in that well enjoyed a more than excellent health: over 80 years old they had no symptoms of old age.

CHAPTER 14

STRESS, MAGNESIUM AND IRIDOLOGY

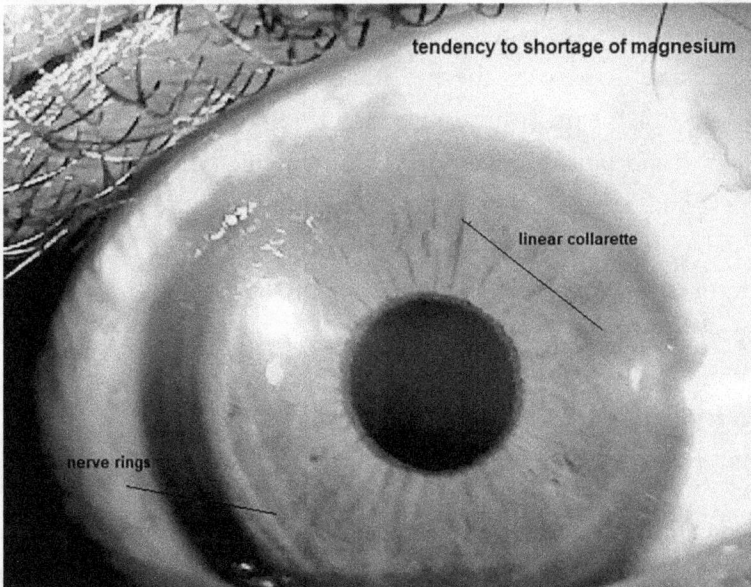

This is a paper that I sent to the organization of a European Integrative Medicine congress for later presentation to the public.

It could be read as an introduction to the potential of iridological analysis, as a preventive tool, as we will later see in the next chapters.

Abstract:

Iridology (Iris Analysis) can offer a little help for better diagnosis of deficiencies of Magnesium (Mg), which is quite common today. Unfortunately, blood tests and the observation of some symptoms is not an accurate way of diagnosing the level of Hypomagnesemia. The analysis of the iris is a very easy and quick method, and with only a photo, a fairly accurate investigation diagnosis can be achieved.

Why is magnesium so important?

Magnesium is found within every cell of the human body and is essential to all living organisms. Over 300 enzymes require magnesium to regulate different biochemical reactions in the body. The mineral controls the activity of the hypothalamic-pituitary-adrenal (HPA) axis, which is the main stress response system. Magnesium levels may play an important role in mood disorders, including stress, anxiety, sadness and depression. All the enzymes that create ATP for energy are dependent on magnesium. Its many functions include helping with muscle and nerve function, regulating blood pressure, and supporting the immune system.

Why is the deficiency so common?

The average healthy adult requires around 300-400 mg of magnesium per day, but magnesium deficiency is one of the most common nutritional deficiencies in adults today (some studies speculate around 70-80 %).

In my observations of pictures of the iris, I obtained a percentage of 25 - 30 %.

Normal magnesium levels are between 0.6-1.1 mmol/L (1.46–2.68 mg/dL) with levels less than 0.6 mmol/L (1.46 mg/dL) defining hypomagnesemia. The causes of hypomagnesemia result from the following:

- ⮎ lack of the right amount of the mineral in the diet,
- ⮎ difficulty of magnesium absorption, due to too fast excretion (eg. excessive sweating)
- ⮎ some other nutrients make problems, a dietary imbalances (eg. too much carbohydrate/alcohol/fatty foods)
- ⮎ stress.

Stress is probably the main factor contributing to this deficiency.

Under some particular conditions of mental or physical stress, magnesium is released from the blood cells and goes into the blood plasma. From there, it's excreted via the urine. This situation creates a condition of new stress in a vicious circle.

Muscle twitches and cramps, sleep and mental disorders, osteoporosis, fatigue and muscle weakness, high blood pressure, and irregular heartbeat could all be signs of Mg deficiency.

How to Identify a Magnesium Deficiency.

Hypomagnesemia can be diagnosed by a medical physical examination, involving checking particular symptoms, examining the medical history, and making a blood test. A blood magnesium level doesn't reveal the amount of magnesium the body has stored in the bones and muscle tissue (99 %) and only a tiny amount of magnesium is normally present in the blood. (1 %)

How Iridology helps.

An easier and simpler method is to observe signs in the iris of the eye of a patient.

Iridology gives interesting information through studying the following signs in the iris.

The nerve rings.

The nerve rings are quite common and easily to observe and they show many different signs of stress like anxiety,depression, and mental disorders. They are named Contraction furrows or Stress rings or Cramps rings. Mostly are circular, but may be concentric arcs or a portion of arc spread throughout the iris. Iridologists think that this sign is strictly related to stress and consequently reveal a shortage of minerals (magnesium) They can be a direct sign (or indirect sign) of depression, chronic fatigue, or difficulties with absorption of calcium, zinc, selenium, magnesium, potassium, vitamin D e vitamin B groups.

These rings, are caused by the constant or prolonged contraction of the dilator muscle (indicating abnormal tension in the sympathetic nervous system and a weakness in the adrenal gland) These signs, can be seen quite often in people with insomnia, sweaty palms, diabetes and other neurological diseases related to stress. Sometimes the signs are inherited or sometimes appear after a long period of life difficulties. The presence of rings usually indicate that a person is a particularly sensitive.

Analysts can determine the level of stress by considering the number and the consistency of the rings. The length, the depth and the color of the rings are factors that can show the severity of the problem.

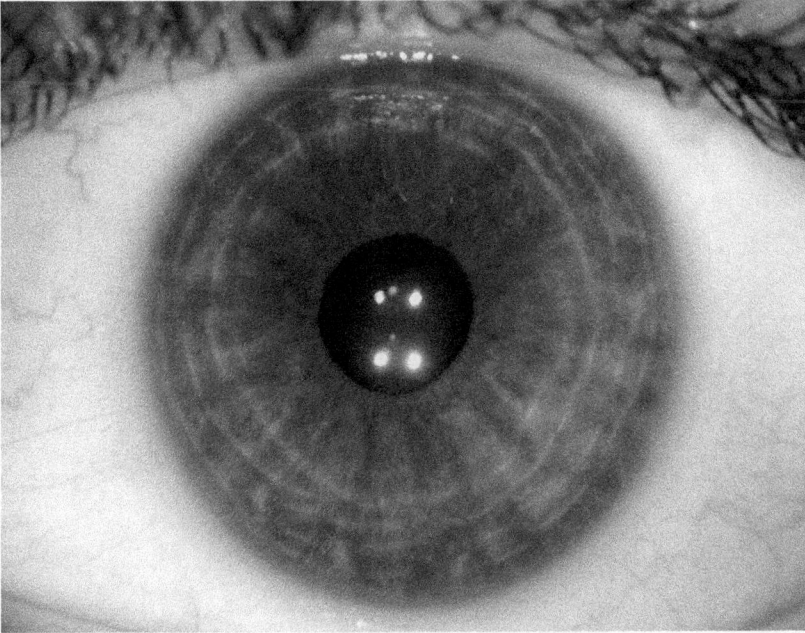

https://www.iriscope.org/iridology-stress-
ringswhatwhyand-the-mean.htm

After the nerve rings there is another sign related more specifically to the tendency of low levels of Mg. This sign is the linearity of the collarette in the area of the north east of the iris.

The collarette.

Roughly one third out from the pupil there is a circular structure, or ring, called the collarette, or ANW (autonomic nerve wreath). This circle, when present more or less, is the most important landmark to observe because it suggests many interesting weaknesses, caused by the imbalance between the sympathetic and parasympathetic nervous systems and may indicate other aspects about the health of the person.

The collarette indicates the intestinal tract, which is separate from all the other organs, glands and structures. It gives an idea of the state of the intestine. It is a kind of border that divides the internal and the external area of the personality. To some extent it can indicate, for example, if a person is introvert or extrovert, calm or particularly reactive.

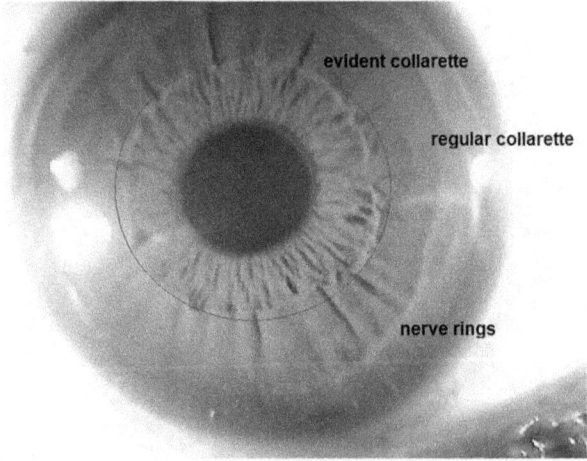

The shape of the collarette is approximately circular (like a ring). Generally it should be like that, but often it assumes a particular shape, irregular in different ways.

One of these irregularities is the presence of straighter sides, so from the ideal shape of a circle , the collarette become more like a polygon.

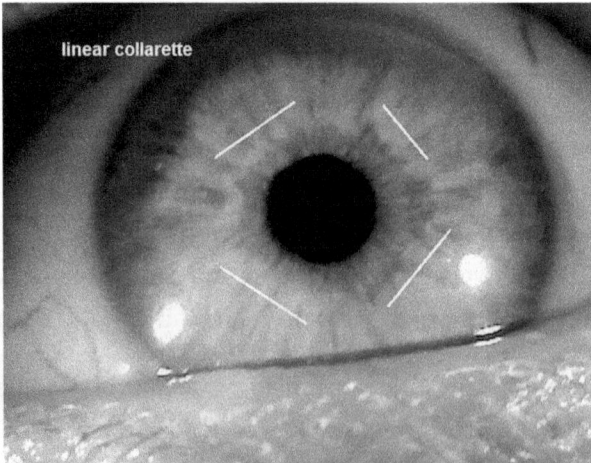

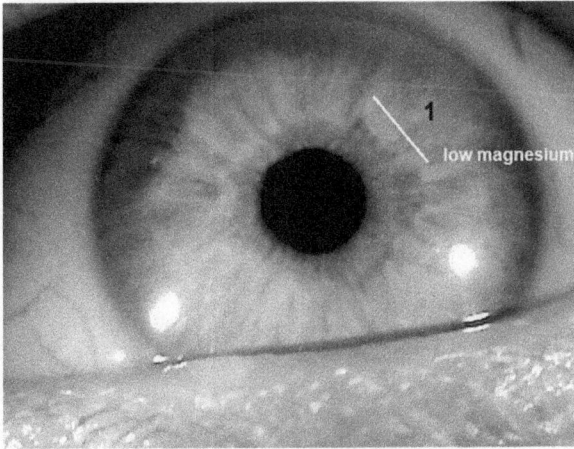

When the linearity is in the area 1, we think a possible shortage of Mg.

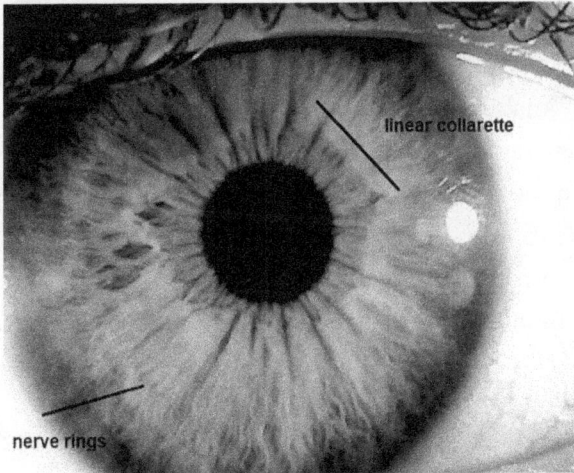

If the two signs, nerve rings and linear collarette, are both present the diagnosis of a shortage of Mg, is more probable.

Conclusion

Iridology can offer a little help for better diagnosis of deficiencies of Magnesium (Mg),

CHAPTER 15

THE IRIS ANALYSIS

Definition:

"Iris Analysis, or Iridology, is a medical technique where characteristics of the iris, such as pattern and color, can be examined to determine information about a person's systemic health. Due to a lot negative health practices when acute situations need to be corrected, alternative health methods and techniques have not been promoted by the medical society...quite frankly...that is not their field."

https://truebetteryou.com/2019/10/21/
health-what-an-iris-analysis-can-reveal/

Iridology is an integrative diagnostic method that is based on the accurate observation of a photo, enlarged, of the iris.

It's a non-invasive, easy, fast and cheap method, which can sometimes highlight some aspects of health that are sometimes unknown, little considered or more difficult to highlight with official diagnostics.

For example, magnesium deficiency, which we will see in the next chapter.

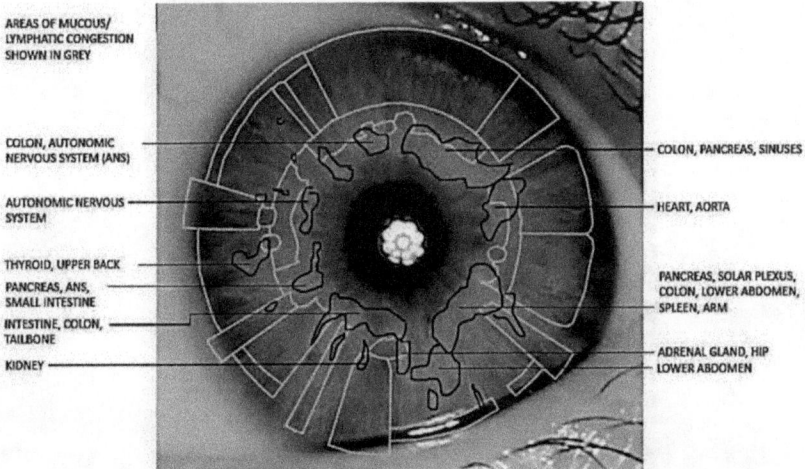

AREAS OF MUCOUS/
LYMPHATIC CONGESTION
SHOWN IN GREY

COLON, AUTONOMIC
NERVOUS SYSTEM (ANS)

AUTONOMIC NERVOUS
SYSTEM

THYROID, UPPER BACK
PANCREAS, ANS,
SMALL INTESTINE
INTESTINE, COLON,
TAILBONE
KIDNEY

COLON, PANCREAS, SINUSES

HEART, AORTA

PANCREAS, SOLAR PLEXUS,
COLON, LOWER ABDOMEN,
SPLEEN, ARM

ADRENAL GLAND, HIP
LOWER ABDOMEN

This figure was uploaded by Mohammad Mahdi Dehshibi
Content may be subject to copyright.

https://www.researchgate.net/publication/291505856_
Iris_the_Picture_of_Health_Towards_Medical_
Diagnosis_of_Diseases_based_on_Iris_Pattern

This topic will be dealt with superficially, in order to give an idea of what it is about, because it is a complex matter. It would take a whole book to describe everything, to be told, also the studies are constantly evolving and every now and then something new is discovered. I hope that I will be able to publish a manual which collect my most interesting experiences, soon.

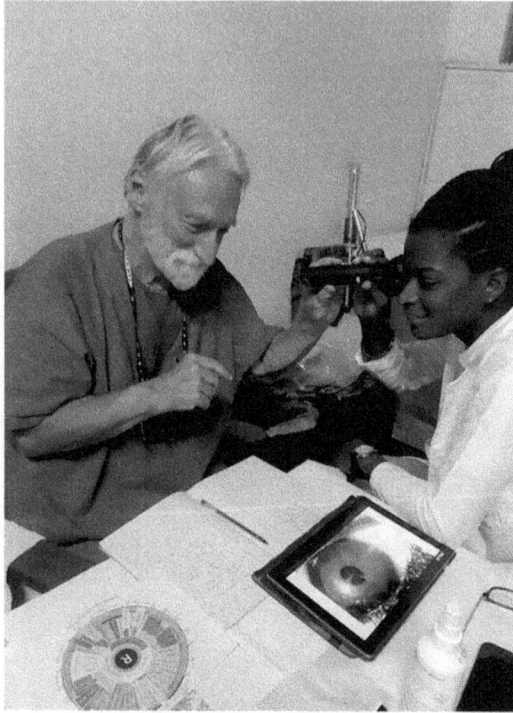

Here I am working at a hospital in Ghana.

Through the observation of the eyes, especially through the irises, it is possible to recognize the current state of health of a patient, past disorders, possible future ones as well as identifying some aspects of the character. At a preventive level it can be a simple survey tool to understand a multitude of curious and interesting elements.

It is a very ancient technique known and used from various ancient civilizations, such as Chinese, Egyptian (1500 BC) and Greek (Hippocrates), we also have traces in Mesopotamia (700 BC).

During 1670, in Dresden in Germany, a doctor named, Philippus Meyens published the first true document in the treatise entitled "Medical Palmistry" ("Medical Phisiognomy") where the characteristics of the iridological signs relating to the condition of the whole organism are described.

But the real birth of this material proper is due (1837) to a young Hungarian boy Ignatz von Peczely (1826-1907), considered the father of modern Iridologia. He was already a curious enthusiast of health-related things and was only 11 years old when observing the iris of an owl, of which he had incidentally broken a paw, he saw a remarkable change in the color of the iris.

In other words, he noticed a black spot in the lower part of the iris, a point that is now considered to be in correspondence with the leg. Intrigued by this event he began to observe and study this strange coincidence. He was very involved with health problems. It was said that he was always sick. As an adult he moved to Vienna and enrolled in the University to study medicine.

Here, he finally had the opportunity to satisfy all his curiosity and began to investigate the variations of the iris according to different diseases. He discovered that every part of his body had a match on the iris.

In 1880, Peczely published his research in the book "Discoveries in the Realms of Nature and the Art of Healing", also drawing the first map.

Almost temporarily, in Sweden, another researcher, Reverend Nils Liljequist, published the results of his first observations on the variation of the color of irises following the intake of chemicals (quinine). One curious thing is that the two researchers drew a fairly similar iridologic map while not being aware of each other's work.

Despite some criticism from official medicine his work was continued and deepened by other researchers both in Europe and in the USA. Dr Bernard Jensen, in California, studied and deepened the subject by publishing the first map in 1950, which is still very popular today.

Recently John Andrews, an English researcher, published several books. (Endocrinology and Iridology). Modern Iridology is its most advanced form of survey with new maps. It's known all over the world and it's always out there giving lectures.

In the next chapters we will see some examples of irises of interest.

How to recognize magnesium deficiency, for example, or a bad circulatory or intestinal situation, or a certain level of stress, or other special cases.

Also in Italy there have been many scholars who have deepened and developed the matter. The most famous is the Franciscan Father Emilio Ratti, doctor, biologist, missionary, expert in natural medicine, later becomes president of the Italian Iridology Association.

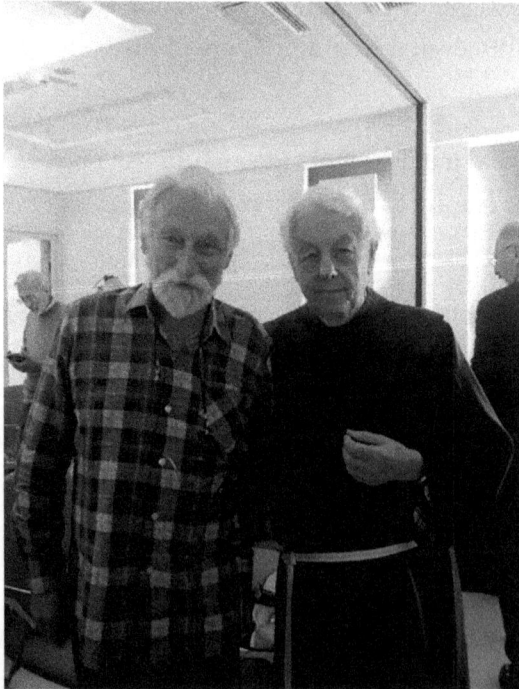

doctor Emilio Ratti and myself at a
recent seminary of Iris Analisis

Then Dr. Rudy Lanza, a founding father of Naturopathy in Italy and director of the school with the same name has also given considerable impetus to the dissemination and study of the iris. He was a Professor of Naturopathy at the Master of Integrative Medicine at the University of Florence, Italy.

What should be observed?

The signs are many and must be evaluated in a broad sense based on their evidence, shape and position.

The color and shades variations, the density of the fibre's bows, rings and their circularity spots gaps and crypts lines and rays of miscellaneous irregularities. Details on the consistency and shape of the collar.

What indications can these signs give us? There are many, to name just a few:

- ➲ The general state of health
- ➲ The reactivity of the autonomic nervous system
- ➲ The level of cellular aging
- ➲ Deficiencies of mineral salts and vitamins
- ➲ The level of stress
- ➲ The level of inflammation
- ➲ Tendency to dysglycemia
- ➲ Tendency to allergies
- ➲ Weakness of the immune system
- ➲ Tendencies to digestive difficulties
- ➲ Functioning of the lymphatic system
- ➲ State of intoxication of the organism

Particularly you can also glimpse the tendency to high cholesterol levels.

The eye does not lie about bad eating habits and a diet rich in trans fats or carbohydrates. High cholesterol and other fats such as triglycerides in arteries often, present as a dull gray ring on the outside of the iris and easily recognizable, even to the naked eye.

Iron deficiency and anemia

Iron deficiency can lead to low energy, weakness, fatigue and anemia, which is the low production of healthy red blood cells. An iron deficiency manifests in the iris as a bright blue ring on the outer edge.

Weakness of particular organs

In correspondence of the various organs we can notice some signs which reveals some events of the past clinical history. This may make you think about future trends.

The lack of magnesium

As we saw in the previous chapter

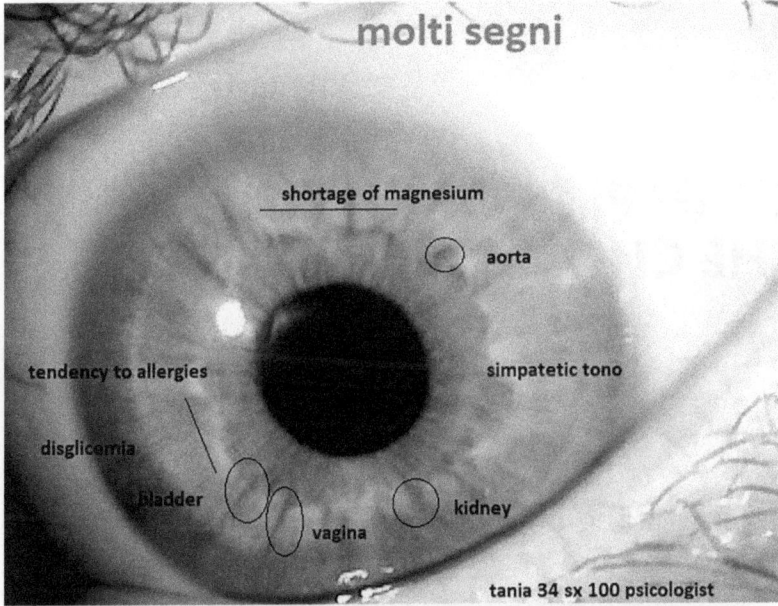

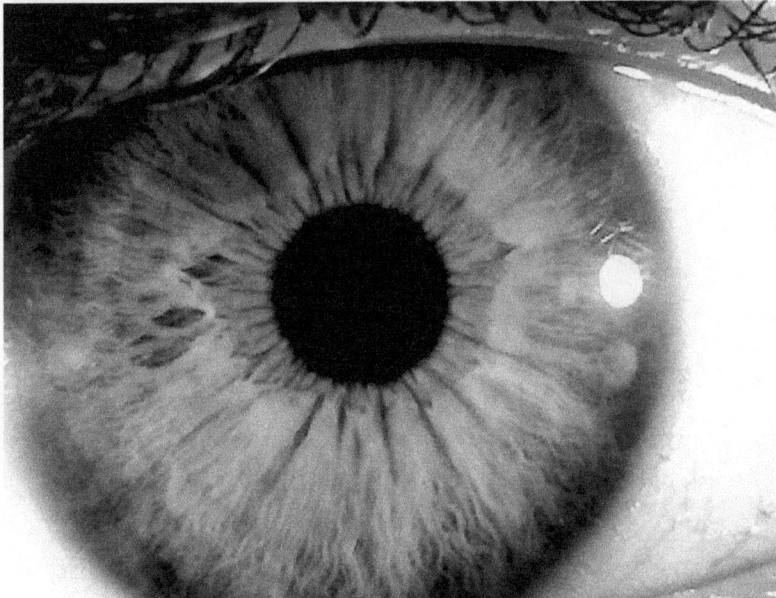

99

CHAPTER 16

EXAMPLES OF IRISES: THE CHOLESTEROL RING.

Premature aging
Biological age

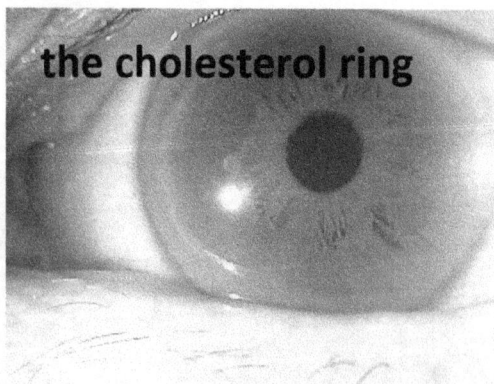

the cholesterol ring

This is a very common sign in people of a certain age, in fact it also has the ring name of **"ring of senility"**, but it also has other names. This could be a clear example of how the ancient wise healers said: ONE sign... a hundred diseases and ONE disease...a hundred signs.

Statistically above 70 years of age, this sign, which occurs with an arc or ring of opaque gray at the edge of the iris, seems to be very common with an incidence of 90% of cases, with a prevalence of men over women and in people of color.

Among the signs that are found in the iris, the cholesterol ring, is one of the easiest to detect, even without sophisticated enlargements, that is, even with the naked eye. This could be an advantage, but the problem is to understand what it could mean. There are at least a dozen hypotheses of possible causes. The common root appears to be a certain circulatory difficulty, presence of fat deposits or minerals such as sodium. One could also say, returning to the definition of senility ring, that it can be a sign of the person's age level. Which is evaluated by considering the consistency and evidence of the sign.

Many people who despite having this obvious sign tell me that with their cholesterol level, after the latest tests, it is normal. So there should be something else behind this sign.

Let's see some other possibilities besides cholesterol.

It could be a sign of excess salt in the diet, an excess of homocysteine or triglycerides, an accumulation of toxins or be a sign of hypertension. Very common in older people.

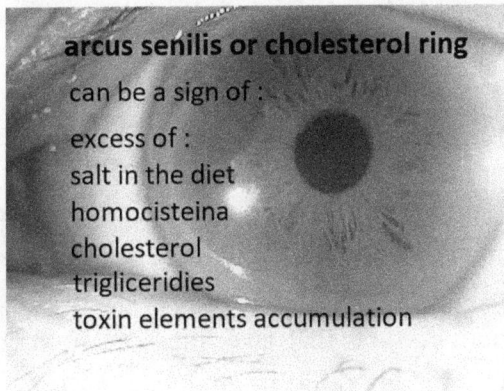

arcus senilis or cholesterol ring

can be a sign of :

excess of :
salt in the diet
homocisteina
cholesterol
trigliceridies
toxin elements accumulation

it could be also a sign of :

Hypertension
Atherosclerosis
poor metabolism of dietary fat

possible shortage of :
potassium
group B vitamins

According to recent research, even a deficiency of vitamins of group B, (B9, B12, B6) seems to be the cause of an excess of homocysteine, which in turn can be decisive. But there can still be some correlations linked to metabolic syndrome, liver, thyroid, and in any case to a careless and unbalanced diet.

Other researchers relate this sign, which they call a ring of determination, to a particular psychological attitude. People, who have a tendency to be inflexible, adamant, convinced of their own ideas, to the excess.

If this sign occurs in younger people, under the age of 50, you might be worried and I would suggest doing some more in-depth investigation of the general state of health. It could be a sign of premature aging, or something else wrong.

Anagraphic and biological age

Some cardiologists argue that a person's true age (biological age) relates to the condition or health of his arteries. Anti-aging medicine, now very fashionable, offers different approaches to this research. There are various theories that take into account various elements but that often have many points in common.

Can you calculate this biological age? Can you guess how far away from the average age? According to some evaluations we may be older or younger than our age. What are the elements to keep under observation?

There are two groups of data, the first group considers measurable, objective data related to physical conditions, such as:

- ➲ abdominal circumference
- ➲ fasting blood sugar
- ➲ blood pressure
- ➲ resting heart rate
- ➲ stress frequency
- ➲ quality/quantity of healty food
- ➲ amount of water consumed
- ➲ level of physical activity

Also recently, a urine-detectable marker (8-oxoGsn) has been discovered that takes into account the oxidation of DNA, which is a true and accurate index of cell aging. (Frontiers in Aging Neuroscience.)

There is, then, a second set of elements to be evaluated which is more difficult to measure, objectively, but perhaps more important. It's more about the mind than the body. Mental health is a good marker of how young we really are. The capacity for imagination, the liveliness of how we relate to the world. The continuous desires to learn and to keep the mind alive and occupied are very positive aspects that would tend to lower this age. Even the good level of the affective world around us can prolong life. Hardly anyone who finds himself alone and depressed does not have a very long life expectancy.

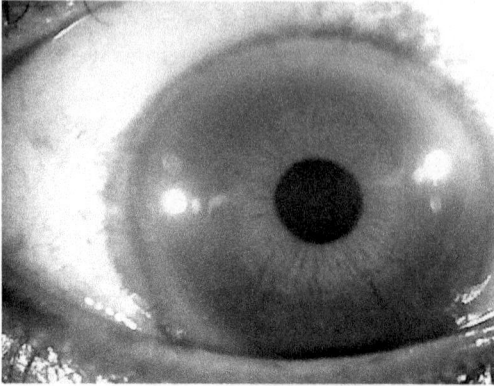

45 year old female
DX
Abdominal c. 105cm
Teacher

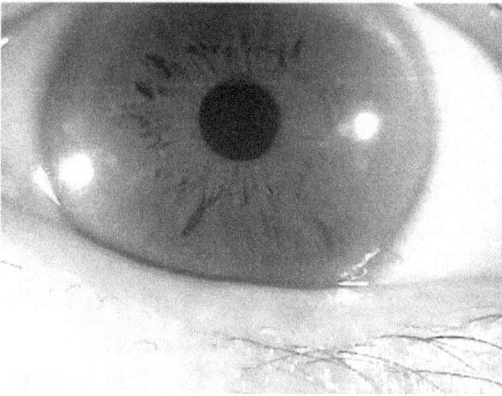

65 year old female.
DX
Abdominal c. 80cm

CHAPTER 17

SOME SPECIAL EXAMPLES OF IRISES

Celibacy

Celiac disease, chronic eating disorder and autoimmune. Interesting research suggests that already at the time of the Romans this disease was known and treated with Chinese medicine with turmeric and gingseng.

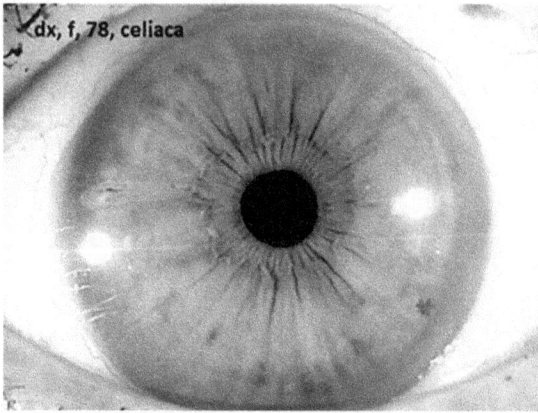

dx, f, 78, celiaca

Stomach reduction or gastrectomy

Middle-aged lady, obese, who underwent gastrectomy surgery, (surgical reduction of the stomach) You notice a sharp change in color in the stomach area.

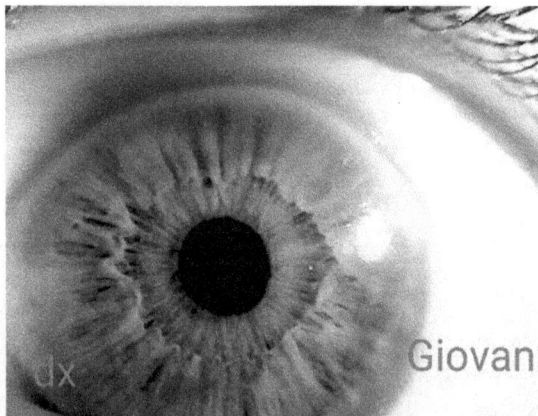

dx   Giovani

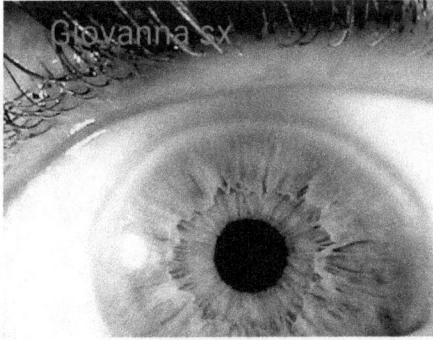

Central eterocromy, Disbiosys

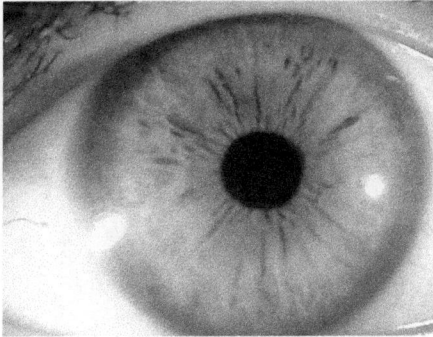

Dialysis

This patient has kidney problems and is undergoing dialysis, which replaces the normal function of the kidney by purifying the blood

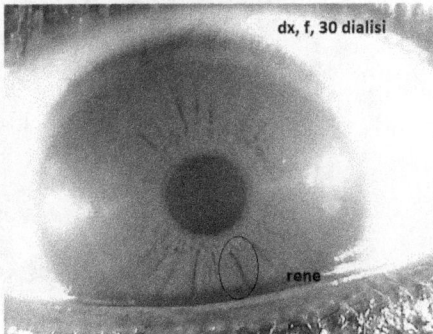

Missing left limb

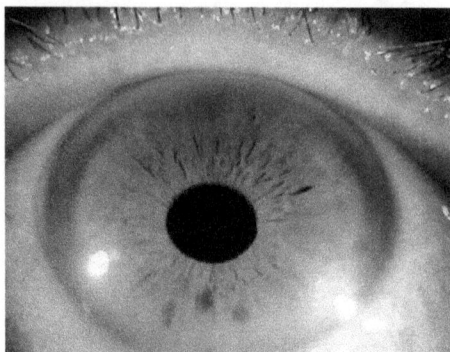

Prediabet

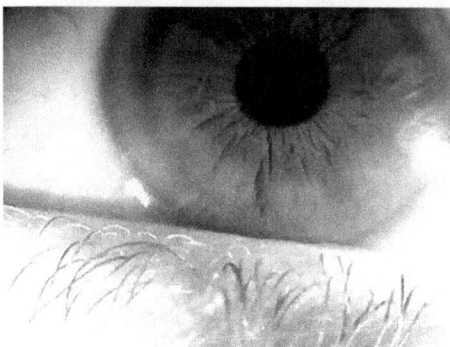

Tinnitus

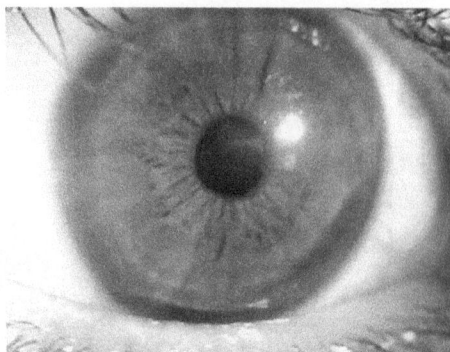

multiple sclerosis

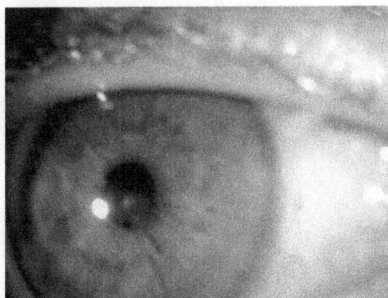

Veganism

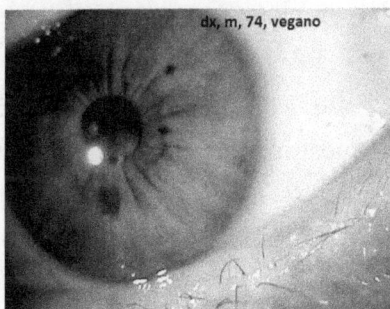

Collapse of the transverse colon

Colon trasverso collassato

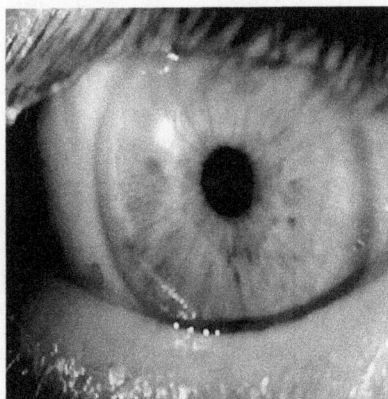

109

CHAPTER 18

THE COLLARETTE

The collarette, also called crown, (ANW, autonomic Nerve wreath) is the most important sign to analyze and the richest information about the psychophysical state of the person.

The collarette represents a line of demarcation between the gastrointestinal part and the other organs. Between the pupillary and the ciliary area. Its structure and conformation can remind us of the shape of the intestine.

You can read in various ways by carefully observing the shape, size, position, consistency, regularity and many nuances.

Among other things it can indicate:

➲ The tone of the autonomic nervous system, its reactivity and vitality
➲ The relationship between the internal and the external world
➲ The efficiency of the immune system

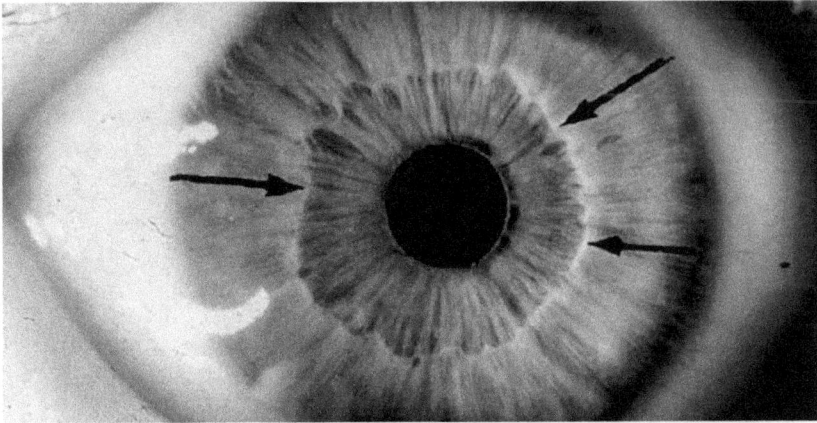

https://www.wellsnaturopathy.com.au/iridology/
an-iridology-snippet-the-collarette/

"The Collarette (also called the Autonomic Nerve Wreath – ANW) is a major Iris landmark. According to the position, shape, colour and its definition an Iridologist can determine specific tendencies associated with bowel function, digestion and nutrient absorption efficiency. It also informs the Iridologist about

a) the state of an individual's nervous system, for instance, whether it is over-reactive (under duress) or under-reactive (fatigued)

b) the personality of the individual, for instance, whether they tend to be more introverted or extroverted and

c) the behavioural tendencies of the individual, for instance, whether they like to be 'in control' and understand the value of discretion or whether they are too willing to share their thoughts, discretion not being their high point. "

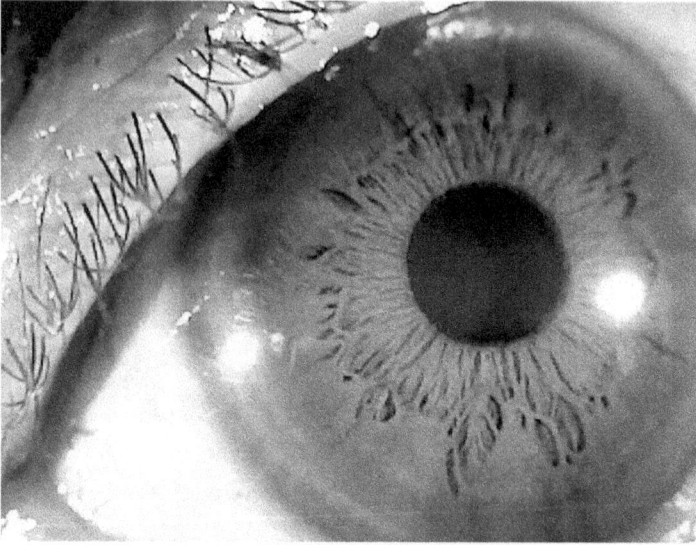

https://www.iridodiagnostics.com/
autonomic-nerve-wreath-the-collarette/

"The autonomic nerve wreath is one of the most important landmarks that an iridologist will analyze. This collarette is well illustrated as the vascular analog for the autonomic nervous system, a circular phenomenon described as representative for the exchange of nutrients and toxic material between the intestinal tract and the body humors. The collarette also serves as an index for the lining of the intestinal tract and autonomic nervous system.

The collarette's circular conformity is a measure of nervous system equilibrium. It suggests a direct link between disturbances in the intestines and peripheral disturbances elsewhere in the body. Thus, it is a very important landmark for the gastrointestinal system, the autonomic nervous system, and the nervous system as a whole.

Collarette wreath distinction, arrangement, and shape all help to identify intestinal activity patterns and reactive character. The ANW broadcasts the response of the system to diversified circumstances of lifestyle, diet and emotional stress. Distinct signs that show these tendencies include crypts, stroma density and central heterochromia, along with radial and contraction furrows.

An obscured Collarette will commonly suggest a condition of toxicity with potential dysfermentias and dysbacteria (dysbiosis). A thickened collarette may indicate toxic materials leaking through intestinal walls, thereby creating a chronic inflammation of the surrounding lymph.

Collarette distention and constriction may also indicate specific types of physical behaviors.

The autonomic nerve wreath is characterized by the following parameters:

- Dimensions of pupillary and ciliary belts
- Pronunciation
- Clarity
- Colour
- Type of form

In the irides of newborns, the autonomic nerve wreath is virtually non-distinguishable; its formation is completed within three to five years of age of these newborns. Usually it looks like an even or broken line, elevated over the deep mesoderm layer where large trabecules form this line. The ANW is a dynamic structure because it can be constricted or increased in volume depending on the continuously changing sizes of the pupillary belt and pupil. For this reason, it is beneficial to carry out biomicroscopic examinations of the autonomic nerve wreath with narrowed pupils, using a bright illumination source. This zone is of great importance for diagnosis, because the collarette is the indicator for the activity of all visceral systems and the reference point for topic diagnostics. It is believed that one can evaluate the functional state of the sympathetic part of the vegetative nervous system by the height and width of the autonomic nerve wreath.

A regular, close to circular form of the autonomic nerve wreath takes place because of the balanced interaction of sphincter and dilator. The sphincter of a pupil has approximately 70-80 separate segments; the widely arranged dilator has no fewer segments. Consequently, in normal function of the autonomic nerve wreath, the harmony in the interaction of the dozens of segments of muscles-antagonists is reached with the assistance of all components of parasympathetic and sympathetic nervous system sections. Good coordination of their work depends on normal harmonic functioning of all internal organs. Any pronounced and prolonged dysfunction of organs, given the pathological viscero-iridal impulses, leads to the disharmony of the autonomous nervous system and, besides the violation of pigment metabolism, to its corresponding deformation.

Under normal conditions, the color of the autonomic nerve wreath corresponds with the iris color, so an increase or decrease of color intensity (local or general) should be considered as pathological symptoms.

Many iridodiagnostic researchers view the autonomic nerve wreath to be tightly connected with many important organs, so pathological signs of this formation are associated with the pathology of the corresponding organs. The roughest sign, indicative of the most severe pathology, is the rupture. The rupture can point to the irreversible pathology of the vegetative nervous system components or hypofunction of the corresponding organs. For example, a rupture in the upper part of the autonomic nerve wreath can point to radix neurological symptoms in the cervical section of the spinal column.

Special signs for the autonomic nerve wreath are typical for certain diseases. There are Russian data that some changes are intrinsic for people with mental diseases. Besides the structural disorganization of iris stroma in the brain projection, local protrusion of the autonomic nerve wreath into this area is most typical of a schizophrenic iridological sign. Some patients have a double protrusion without ruptures, a "horns" symptom, while others have a protrusion that violates autonomic nerve wreath integrity.

Local drawing out of the autonomic nerve wreath indicates the pathology of an organ for which the projection of such drawing is directed.

Local drawing out at the lateral departments of both irises is observed in patients with cardiac pathology (post-infarction cardiosclerosis, rheumatic failures, hypertrophy of the left ventricle). The connection among location, extent of autonomic nerve wreath protrusion and hypertension in certain heart cavities was previously studied in Russia. On the left iris, local protrusion in the heart projection is three times more common than in the right. The light extent of autonomic nerve wreath deformation corresponds with the compensated hypertrophy if myocardium, average, with the initial stages of the dilation, rough, with pronounced dilation. It is supposed that a rupture in this area, which takes place very rarely, is a symptom of aneurysm formation.

Ptosis of the abdominal organs is accompanied with specific changes in the autonomic nerve wreath. Insignificant ptosis of the transverse colon, which can have no clinical manifestations, is reflected in iridology by the flattening of the autonomic nerve wreath in the upper departments.

The rough ptosis of the transverse colon with the prolapse of the abdomen cavity organs is associated with the pronounced flattening of the autonomic nerve wreath, not only in the upper part, but also in the lower one. In such cases it is necessary to distinguish the lower flattening from that drawn in the autonomic nerve wreath in the

"5.00 – 7.00" sector, which takes place in people with an ulcerous disease of the duodenum. To be more precise, it is the marking of the inherited inclination to gastroduodenitis, duodenum ulcer.

In bronchial asthma, changes in the autonomic nerve wreath take place in the area of the lungs-bronchi, in atherosclerosis of the lower extremities in the area of the brain and pelvic organs. Strictures of the transverse colon can be associated with the local pronounced drawing in of the autonomic nerve wreath, diverticulum of the large intestine with some small local drawing out. Such signs can be multiplied in diverticulosis. Importance is attached to the violation of the ratio between the sizes of pupillary and ciliary belts (in the normal state, radial dimensions of the ciliary belt is one-half to two-thirds from the iris' radius). Deviation from these data is often a symptom of the nervous system and digestive tract diseases. If computer processing is not available and estimation of the relative dimensions is difficult, the conditional subdivision into the circular areas is applied. According to recent investigational data, besides the abovementioned symptoms of changed form, the structure and color of the autonomic nerve wreath, the type of its reaction to different kinds of irritants, and the so-called associated reactions all seem to be very important issues."

CHAPTER 19

SOME DIFFERENT COLLARETTES TYPES

Restricted
....

Enlarged
....

Absent/no evidence/tiny
....

Hypertrophic
....

Squared
....

Polygonal
....

The collarette , also called crown, (ANW, autonomic Nerve wreath) is the most important sign to analyze and the richest information about the psychophysical state of the person.

The collaratte represents a line of demarcation between the gastrointestinal part and the other organs. Between the pupillary and the ciliary area. Its structure and conformation can remind us of the shape of the intestine.

You can read in various ways by carefully observing the shape, size, position, consistency, regularity and many nuances.

Among other things it can indicate:

the tone of the autonomic nervous system and its reactivity and vitality

the relationship between the internal and the external world

The efficiency of the immune system

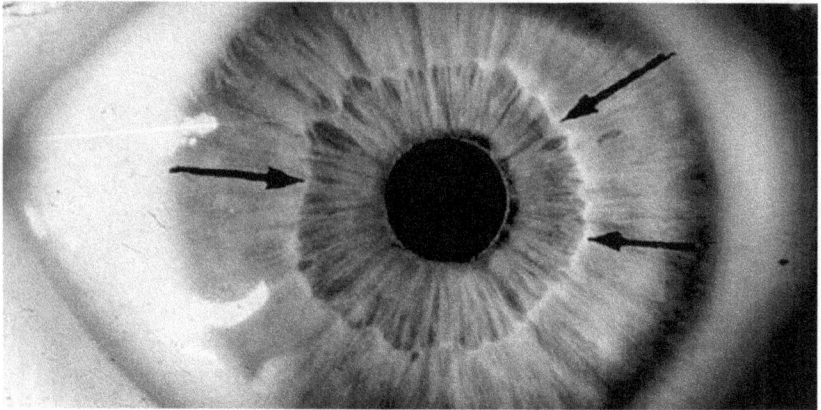

https://www.wellsnaturopathy.com.au/iridology/
an-iridology-snippet-the-collarette/

Another definition:

"The Collarette (also called the Autonomic Nerve Wreath – ANW) is a major Iris landmark. According to the position, shape, colour and its definition an Iridologist can determine specific tendencies associated with bowel function, digestion and nutrient absorption efficiency. It also informs the Iridologist about

    a)   the state of an individual's nervous system, for instance, whether it is over-reactive (under duress) or under-reactive (fatigued)

b) the personality of the individual, for instance, whether they tend to be more introverted or extroverted and

c) the behavioural tendencies of the individual, for instance, whether they like to be 'in control' and understand the value of discretion or are whether they are too willing to share their thoughts, discretion not being their high point

We see now six types of collar:

Narrow, enlarged, absent, hypertrophic, Squared and Poligonal with their peculiarities...

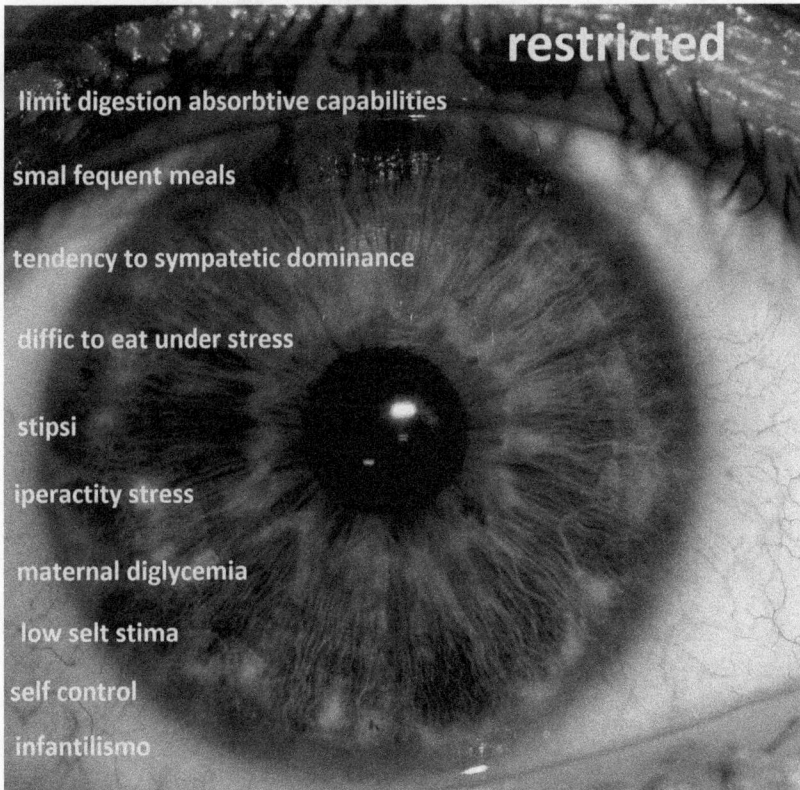

restricted

limit digestion absorbtive capabilities

smal fequent meals

tendency to sympatetic dominance

diffic to eat under stress

stipsi

iperactity stress

maternal diglycemia

low selt stima

self control

infantilismo

The Restricted collarette.

It can be considered narrow when its diameter is less than one third of the total width of the iris.

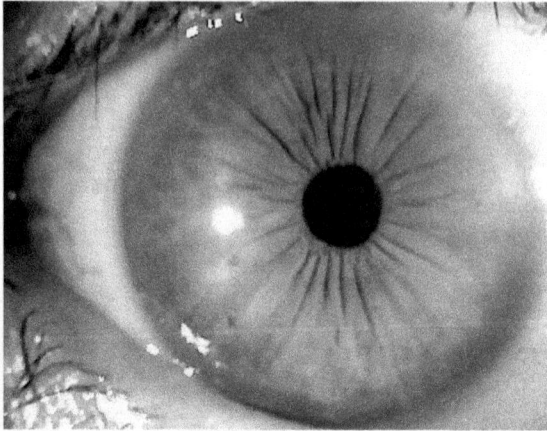

This type of collar could indicate:

strong tendency towards the sympathetic nervous system

limited capacity of digestive absorption

tendency to prefer frequent meals

difficulty eating under stress

stress-induced hyperactivity

low self-esteem and insecurity

mother-induced dysglycemia

constipation, hard and dark stools

self-control, introversion

tendency to close in on oneself to defend oneself from the outside

distended/enlarged collarette

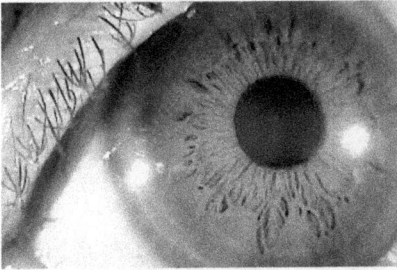

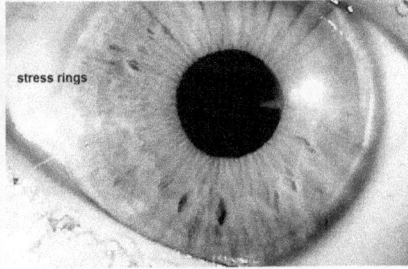

stress rings

these individuals often have a large appetite, tending to:

dilated and irritable colon

good eater, desire to live,

extroversion, generosity

empathy towards the outside world

dispersive difficulties in storing energy

slow transit

bad nutrient absorption

flautolence, costipation

weak tonus of the tract

lack of innervation of the musculature

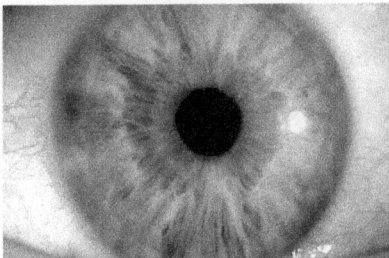

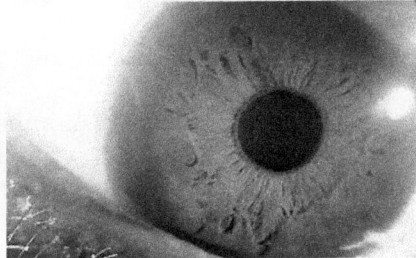

dilated and irritable colon
good eater, desire to live,
extroversion, generosity
empathy towards the outside world
dispersive difficulties in storing energy
slow transit
bad nutrient absorption
flautolence, costipation
weak tonus of the tract
lack of innervation of the musculature

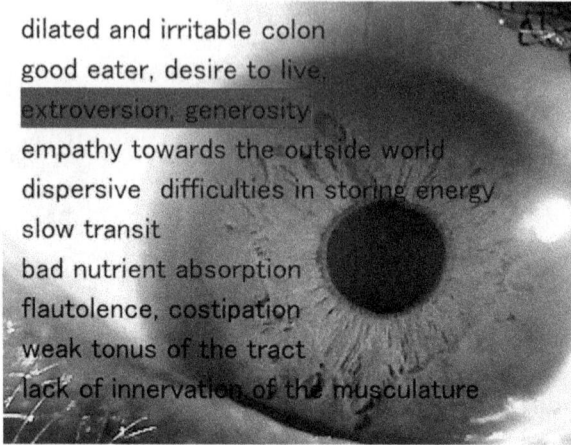

Absent Collarette

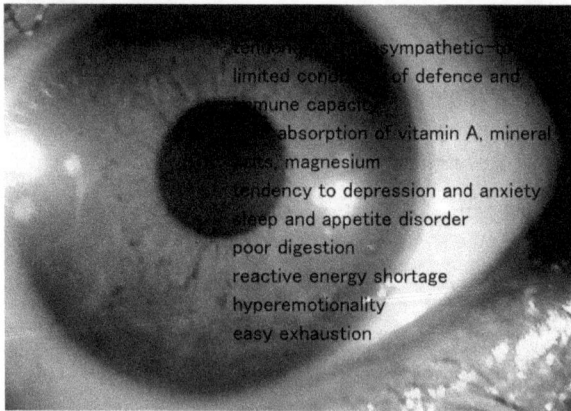

tension   sympathetic-to
limited con   of defence and
mune capaci
absorption of vitamin A, mineral
magnesium
tendency to depression and anxiety
sleep and appetite disorder
poor digestion
reactive energy shortage
hyperemotionality
easy exhaustion

it may indicate:

tendency to parasympathetic-tone

limited conditions of defence and immune capacity

poor absorption of vitamin A, mineral salts, magnesium

tendency to depression and anxiety

sleep and appetite disorder

poor digestion

reactive energy shortage

hyperemotionality

easy exhaustion

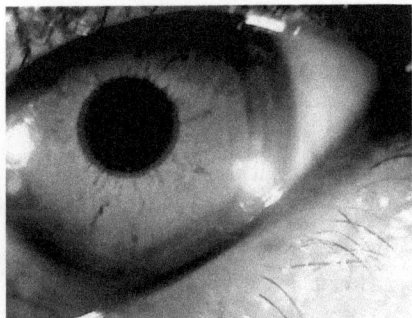

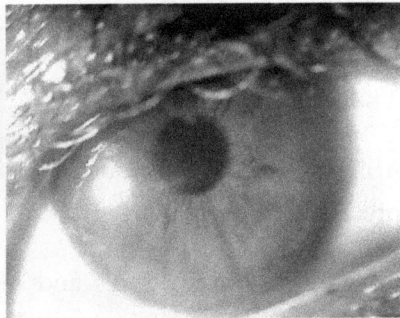

Hypertrophic

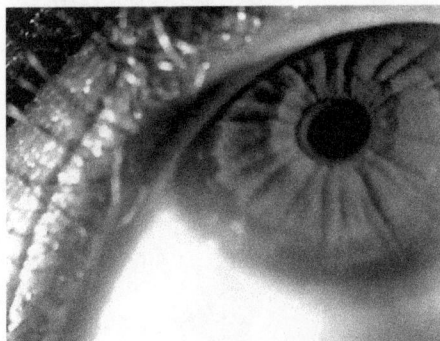

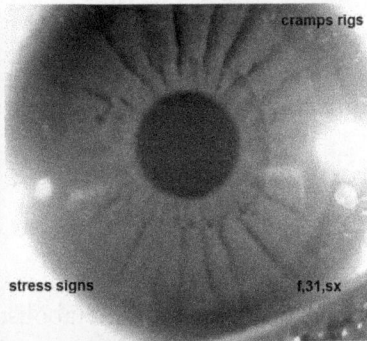

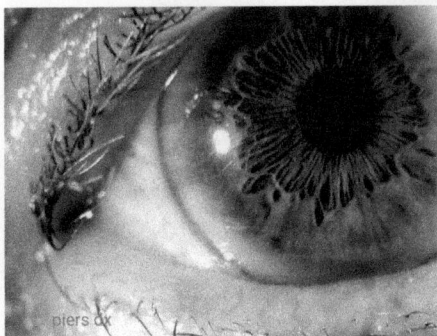

123

The hypertrophic ring can be a sign of:

a predisposition to hyperthymia.

overreaction to physical and psychic stimuli.

Exuberance with energy,

This kind of people can be anxious, impatient, hypersensitive.

They can suffer from:

hypertension with headaches, tinnitus, dizziness, with increased predisposition for heart attacks.

uricemic disorders, lipids and regarding carbohydrate metabolism, possible allergic pathologies, arthrosis diseases.

simpatetic-tone

nervous irritability

intestinal lymph node congestion

compromised immune system

Exuberant with energy

disorders of calcium metabolism

They're anxious, impatient, hypersensitive.

Often, these pronounced collarettes can take on a square, polygonal, double, very irregular and linear shape with many variations

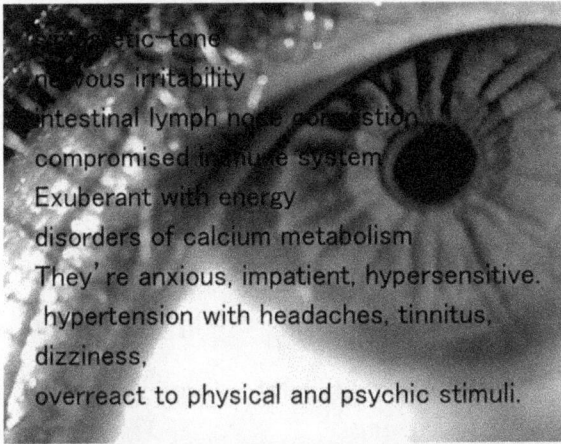

etic-tone
nervous irritability
intestinal lymph node congestion
compromised immune system
Exuberant with energy
disorders of calcium metabolism
They're anxious, impatient, hypersensitive.
hypertension with headaches, tinnitus,
dizziness,
overreact to physical and psychic stimuli.

Squared collarette

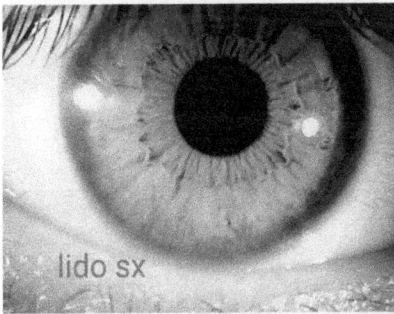

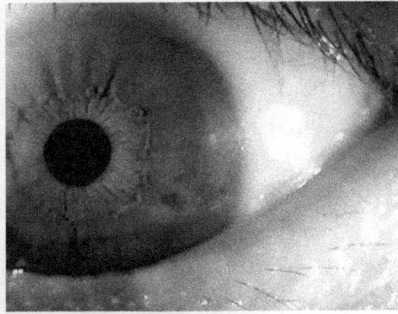

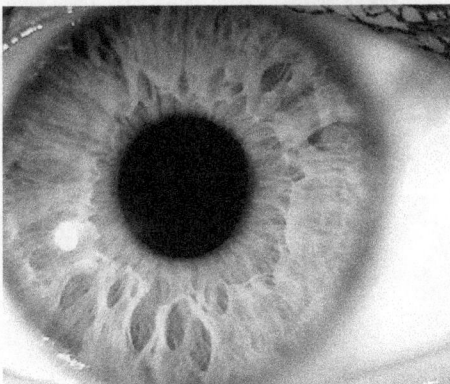

lido sx

Square collar

It is found in those people who have:

certain predisposition to intestinal diseases

a bad intestinal absorption

slow transit

dysglycemia

tendency to respiratory, cardiac and sexual problems

Anabolic metabolic defect: difficulty in forming proteins

normally visible in one eye, if right inherited from father,

left from mother

often hypertrophic

Poligonal Collarette

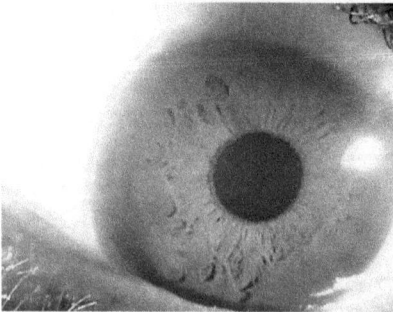

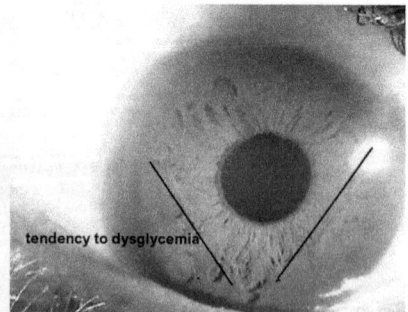

tendency to dysglycemia

CHAPTER 20

OTHER SPECIAL SIGNS:

Radii Solaris

Cramp Rings

Lymphatic rosary

Gastric ring

Heterochromia

Connective weakness

They are folds, quite frequent, due to the contraction of the iris and can have different meanings. They can be of two different types. Those that start from the collar, also called minor, indicate neuro-vegetative disorders influenced by both the digestive system, toxins and parasites, and the hormonal system. If they are concentrated in the cerebral area they can indicate disorders of attention, memory and concentration. If they start from the pupil margin, called major, they could indicate psycho-physical exhaustion, headaches and dizziness, and even insomnia.

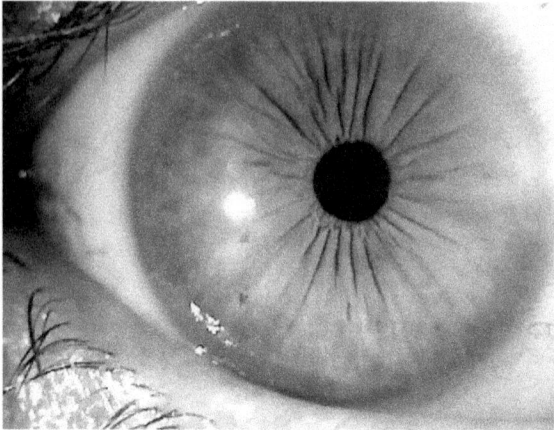

More generally we can say that they are a sign of:

- ➲ Neurovegetative dystonia
- ➲ Insufficient toxin drainage
- ➲ Anxiety, depression and stress
- ➲ Headache and dizziness
- ➲ Difficulty in concentration and memory
- ➲ Poor circulation, phlebitis, hemorrhoids
- ➲ Viscular spasms

Cramp rings

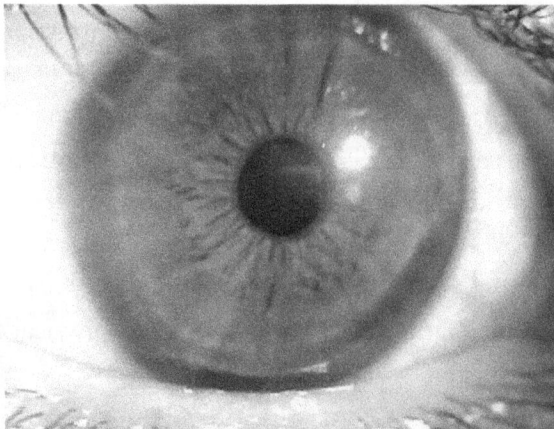

128

This is also a fairly frequent sign and can have many different interpretations, of which the most widely accepted is to indicate a high general level of stress. These arches are supposed to be due to the continuous contraction of the pupil as a result of the rapid shift from the sympathetic to the parasympathetic system. Their consistency, number, and location must be evaluated in order to give a more precise assessment of their significance.

They may therefore be an indication of:

- ⮑ Spasmophilia
- ⮑ Mind body imbalance
- ⮑ Magnesium deficiency
- ⮑ Deficiency of B vitamins
- ⮑ Difficulty in retaining or absorbing minerals
- ⮑ Predisposition to insomnia
- ⮑ Chronic fatigue

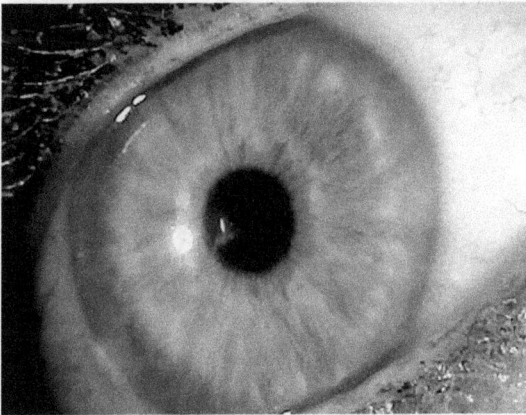

Lymphatic Rosary

Very common in blue iridescents is the presence of the so-called lymphatic rosary or corollary (small white spots, like flakes, arranged in a crown in the periphery).

This sign characterizes the type of the hydrogen subgroup of lymphatic irides. It is thought to be an indication of deposition of calcium salts in connective tissue and joints with accumulation of moisture. In other words, the lymphatic system is not functioning too well. Lymphatic circulation also relies on muscle contraction and therefore to avoid congestion it is suggested to insist on adequate physical activity.

It may be an indication of:

- High hypersensitivity of the skin (eczema, urticaria)
- High sensitivity to climatic variations (humidity)
- Tendency to metereopathies and neuralgias
- Deposition of uric crystals in the myelin sheath with neuralgia
- Tendency to nervous irritability (variable mood)

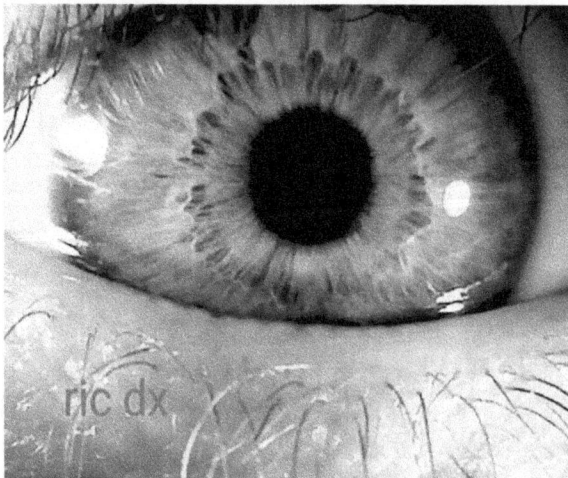

The gastric ring (stomach ring)

It is the first ring that surrounds the pupil. It is often seen very well in people with blue eyes. It gives us an indication of the general condition of the stomach. If this sign is not present we can assume that the stomach is in good balance and everything is in order. In dark or mixed irises this area is often covered by pigment and therefore is not visible or distinguishable. If it is present, in general, it can be assumed that we are in a situation of poor digestion or limited absorption of nutrients. In particular three different situations can occur depending on the color.

If the color is white or light, we assume a situation of acidity (hyperchloridia), if dark we are in the opposite case (hypochloridia), if it has a color tending to orange we assume a tendency to poor metabolism of sugars.

Heterochromia

This is also a very common sign. They are shades or variations of color of various types. Sectoral, ring and central, which are the most common.

Heterochromia is called complete when it affects the entire iris (heterochromia with respect to the other iris); complete heterochromia indicates a non-perfect psychophysical harmony.

Sectoral heterochromia concerns a particular area of the iris, indicating a constitutional weakness or pathological predisposition of the organs corresponding to the heterochromic area.

The central heterochromia is located in the area of the intestine and therefore this is the area concerned. The indications can be many:

- Excessive toxin load
- Intestinal dysbiosis
- Hepatobiliary disorders
- Glandular disorders, pancreas (brown)
- Diabetic / dysglycemic tendency

- ⮑ Problems with parents (orange)
- ⮑ Anxiety affecting digestive system
- ⮑ Hyperprolactinemia
- ⮑ Drug abuse, alcohol, smoking
- ⮑ Food intolerances
- ⮑ Essential fatty acids deficiency
- ⮑ Lack of adequate exercise
- ⮑ Excess carbohydrates

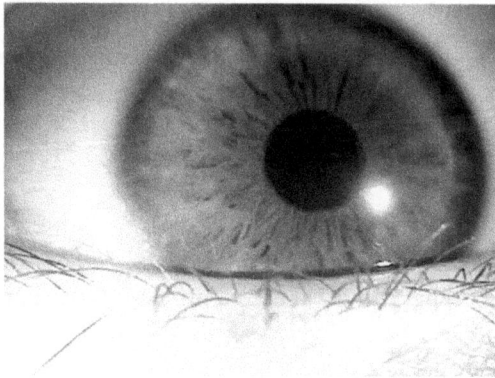

Connective tissue weakness

People with this type of iris often have some ligamentous laxity and possible vitamin C deficiency

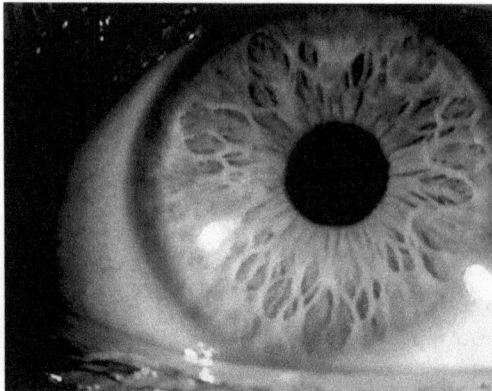

CHAPTER 21

AURICULAR THERAPY

Definition, history, functioning

The treatment, reflex and functional points

The fields of application, benefits.

Examples

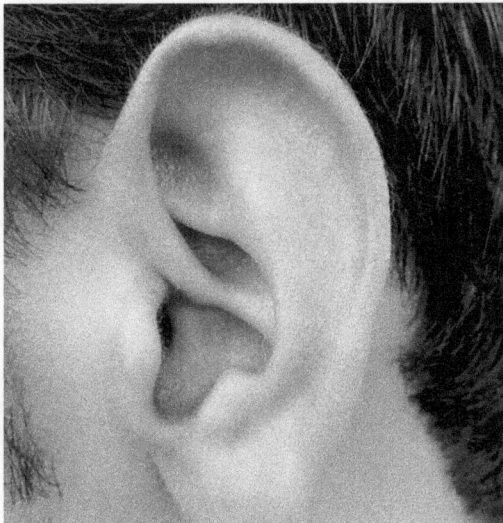

www.AcupunctureProducts.com

D iscipline belonging to integrative medicine that uses the auricle for diagnostic and therapeutic purposes.

Auricular Therapy Reflex

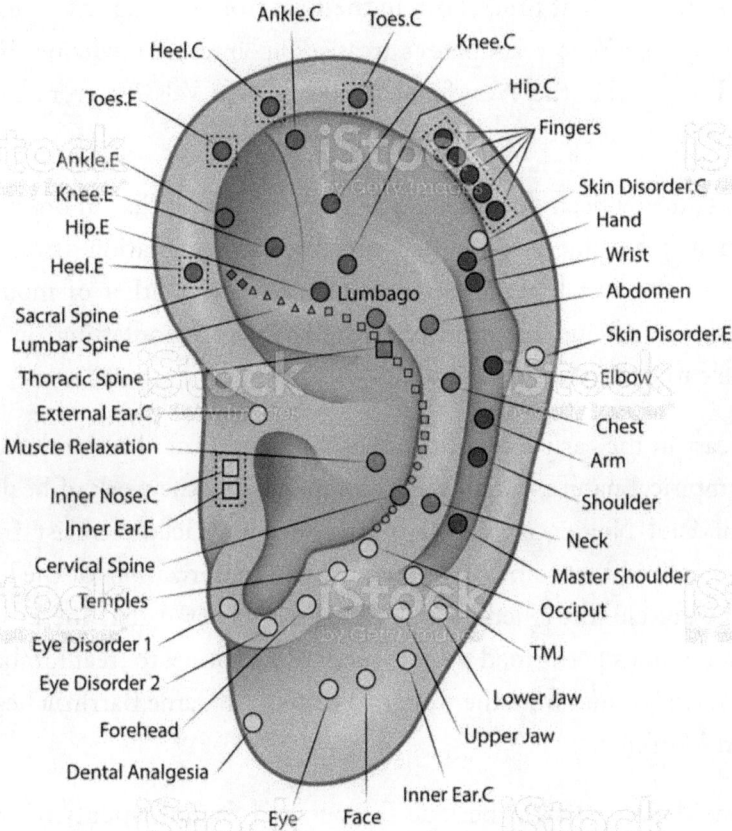

Due to the studies by Paul Nogier MD a French acupuncturist, carried out in the 1950s, the discovery was made that the pinnae are home to reflex points and areas whose stimulation can affect the functions of the entire organism.

We know, for example, that the auricle is innervated by important cranial nerves, including the vagus nerve. When the point from where the nerve passes is stimulated, the stimulation is reflected on nerve centers which control important vital functions such as heartbeat, digestion, respiration, sense of hunger, mood, and sleep-wake rhythm.

The study of the auricle for therapeutic purposes has been handed down since ancient times, both in the East from the ancient Chinese (Neijing: the Yellow Emperor's treatise on "internal medicine, 500-300 B.C.) and in the West from Hippocrates to Valsalva, from Colla to Borelli.

It has already been documented in Ancient Egypt, that in order for women to become infertile they underwent cauterization of certain areas of the auricle. Later, even Hippocrates, the father of modern Western medicine, reported performing micro bloodletting on the auricle to treat male impotence.

At least in the early days, this medical practice was characterized by its empirical nature, which was accompanied by the work of healers. Until Paul Nogier, a general practitioner and acupuncturist from Lyon noticed that some of his patients had cauterizations at the level of the auricle. Intrigued by this fact, he discovered that these were cauterizations performed by non-medical personnel to treat lumbago and sciatalgia and were the work of a certain Madame Barrin, a healer from Marseille.

Soon Madame Barrin became famous and found patients to treat with ease, all over southern France, because this system worked incredibly well. As the story goes, she received this secret from her father. He learnt it from a Chinese mandarin who wanted to repay him for his hospitality.

The cauterized point was not yet known in acupuncture, because the classical points on the various meridians stop around the ear. Despite the temptation to reject the method, Dr. Paul Nogier wanted to find an explanation immediately, as it was normal at the time because it came from street healers. It is still the case today. He began to wonder if there any comparisons could be found between certain areas of the ear and peripheral organs.

One day he was reminded of the phrase so often uttered by Dr. Amathieu who taught him spinal manipulations:

"Sciatica is a problem of the 5 lumbar vertebrae". It begins to dawn on him that the spot cauterized by Mrs. Barrin may correspond, approximately, to the fifth lumbar vertebra.

The anthelix, the part of the ear, which forms a fold in the middle of the pinna, could therefore correspond to the spine. Then, by dint of looking at her patients` ears, she finds that the ear resembles a fetus folded in on itself, its head pointing downward.

https://tcm-project.com/auriculotherapy-101/

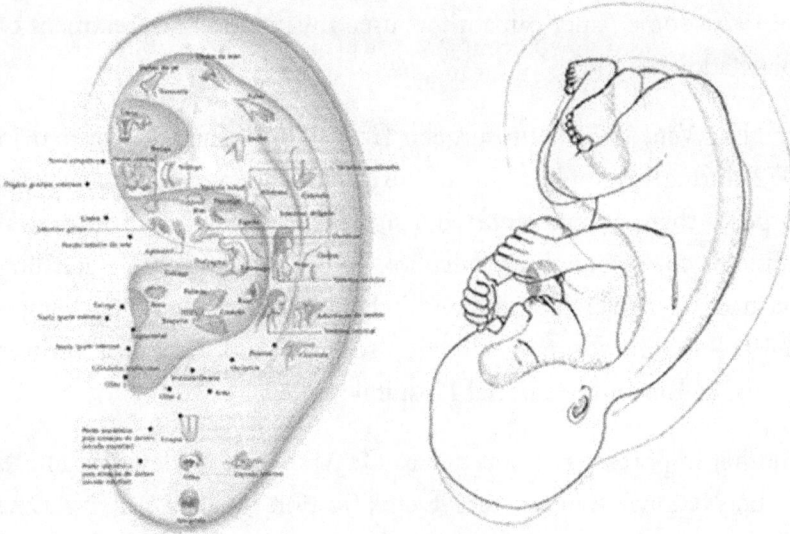

He then finds that when patients complain about the lower back region, the corresponding point is painful to pressure.

The same technique is then used on all patients who complain about the back. It is not slow to point out that the region located a little lower on the anthelix is in correspondence with the back and that even lower still finds areas in relation to cervicalgia. Thus the anthelix is in reverse, in perfect analogy with the spine. More so, its different incisure seems to mark separations between the cervical, dorsal and lumbar vertebral zones.

His work was published in 1957 and gave some scientific merit to this method.

The work attracted much interest from the scientific world around the globe. In China, Nogier's work was reworked and deepened through old knowledge in the field of Traditional Chinese Medicine (TCM). This led to the development of a Chinese auricular map (Shanghai College of TMC in '74) that differed from Nogier's in some elements. The method was named Auricular Acupuncture. In the 1970s some American authors used this method for treatment of opiate addiction.

Dr HL Wen, 1972 neurosurgeon from Hong Kong, discovered in 1972 during his applications of auricular acupuncture for analgesic purposes that patients reported a significant decrease in withdrawal problems to various drugs (alcohol, opium, cocaine). This startling fact had a considerable echo and helped publicize auricular therapy. In 1974 a clinic for drug addiction recovery and detoxification was opened at Lincoln Memorial Hospital in New York.

Another important step was due to Dr. M. Smith of New York, head of the National Acupuncture Detoxification Association (NADA) who described a protocol (1985), for the treatment of drug abuse. Later, in 1992, Prof. JS Han and his colleagues at the Neuroscience Research Institute of Peking University did the same.

So this technique is appreciated and known from East to West, although some differences remain, in fact today there are still maps of Chinese points and French points.

How points can be treated.

There are various methods to treat auricular points, today, first and foremost acupuncture: either filiform needles (kept in place for a few minutes) or dwelling needles (kept in place for a few days) are used: this is strictly a medical method. But there are also other less invasive methods, which can be considered to all intents and purposes within the competence of a naturopath:

Massage: a convenient self-treatment

Pressure: Also to assess the sensitivity of different points, those that are more sensitive or painful, need to be treated with more care and consistency.

Application of vaccaria seed patches: these small seeds are used and applied to the points and kept in place for a few days, taking care to press them several times a day (as appropriate). The application of vaccaria seeds is absolutely safe, they never cause adverse reactions (alleys, ulceration): however, sometimes a stimulated spot can be very painful, in case you cannot bear this pain for a long time you can safely remove the seed by peeling off the patch.

Laser: a laser beam is aimed at points or areas.

Electrostimulation: prongs connected to an electrical circuit are used to stimulate the points; a mild, low-intensity current discharge is felt, usually easily tolerated.

Application of magnetic microspheres (gold or silver plated): these are a more effective alternative to vaccaria seeds because they act continuously without having to be manipulated.

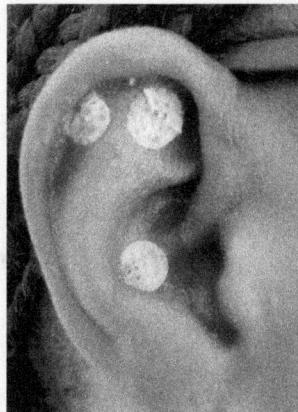

What are the points to be treated?

In general, 2 different types of points are distinguished:

1) **Reflex points** of organs or body parts: heart, stomach, spleen, kidney

2) **Functional points:** points that do not have precise anatomical correspondences which are used for specific purposes or general rebalancing. There are about 20 of them.

Reflex points

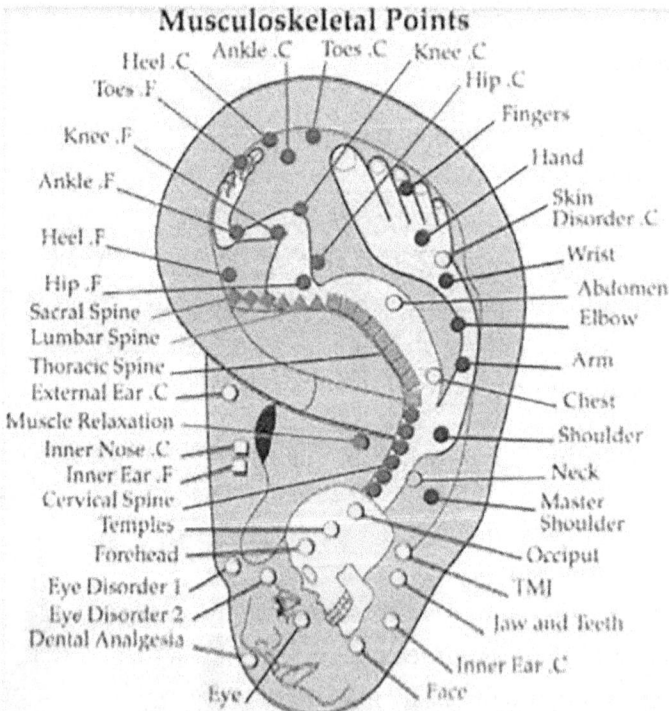

Musculoskeletal Points

Re-printed with permission of Terrence Oleson PhD

Functional points

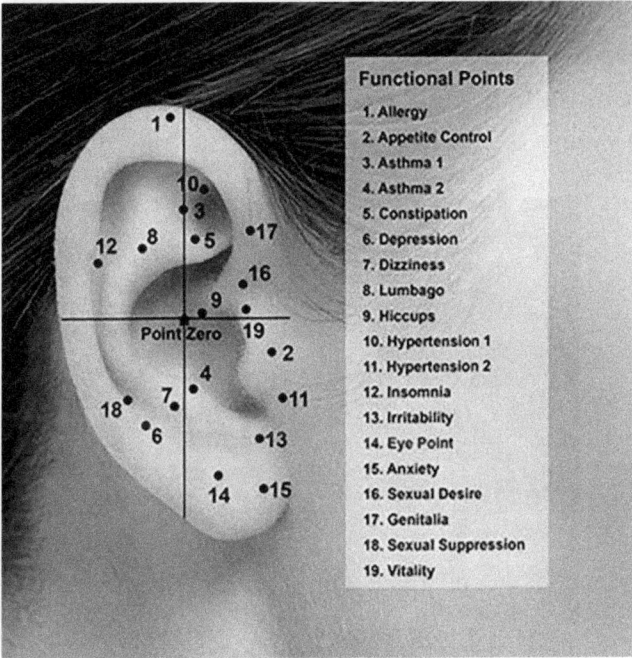

Functional Points

1. Allergy
2. Appetite Control
3. Asthma 1
4. Asthma 2
5. Constipation
6. Depression
7. Dizziness
8. Lumbago
9. Hiccups
10. Hypertension 1
11. Hypertension 2
12. Insomnia
13. Irritability
14. Eye Point
15. Anxiety
16. Sexual Desire
17. Genitalia
18. Sexual Suppression
19. Vitality

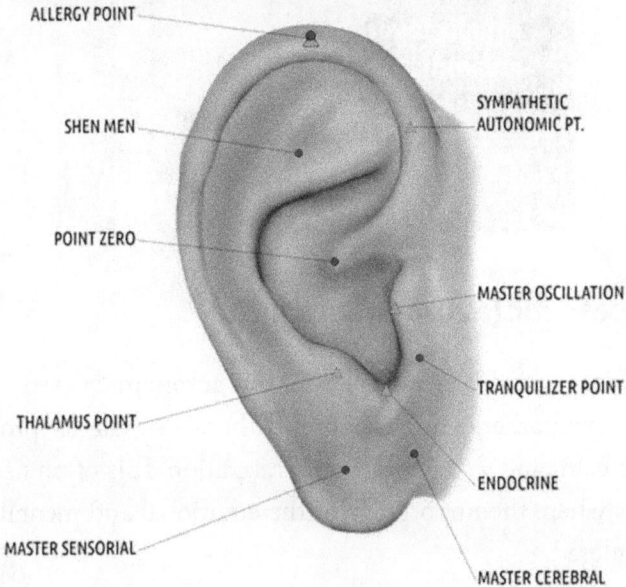

Let's look at the first three most important functional points

Shenmen:

located in the upper part of the auricle, in the triangular basin, is the general psychic balancing point, has sedative, pain-relieving, anti-inflammatory action. It is the **most** important and also the most used point, in various therapies.

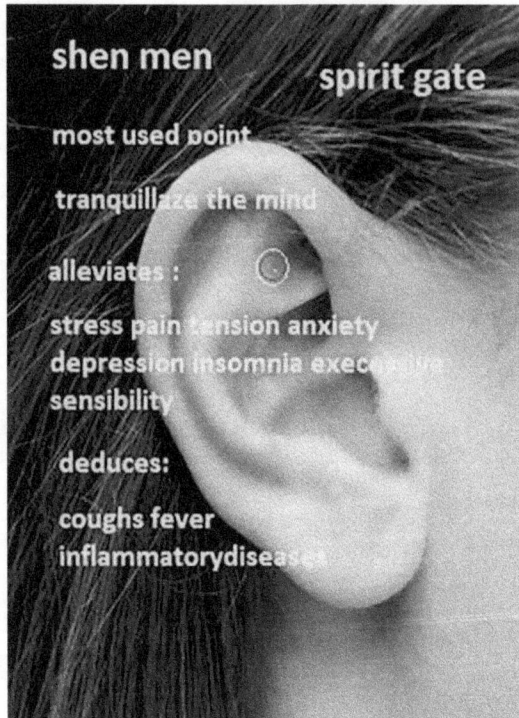

Sympathetic (autonomic point):

located high on the helix. It balances our autonomic nervous system between sympathetic and parasympathetic, so as to promote a return to calm and a state of general relaxation. It is often used in all therapies where the importance of the emotional and mental aspects are considered.

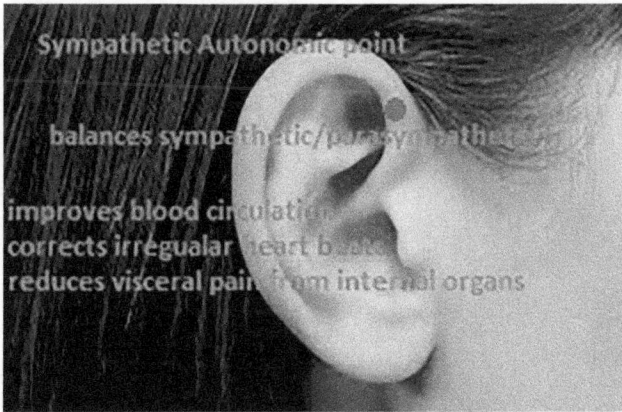

Point Zero:

It is the geometric and physiological center of the entire auricle. (It would correspond to the navel of the fetus). It brings the whole body toward homeostasis, producing a balance of energy, a balance of hormones, and a balance of brain activity.

It also supports the actions of the other points. "Stimulating this point also acts on the vagus nerve, which is next in this area.

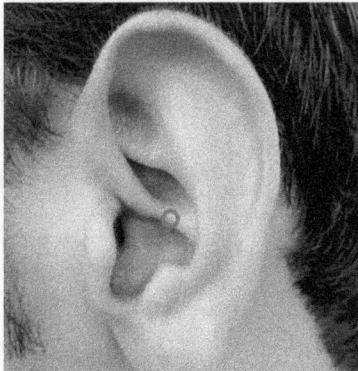

Just the combination of stimulation of these three points induces a certain sense of relaxation with considerable stress reduction and is already a classic therapy.

143

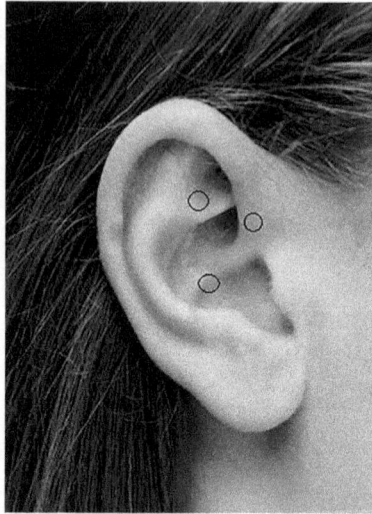

Fields of application

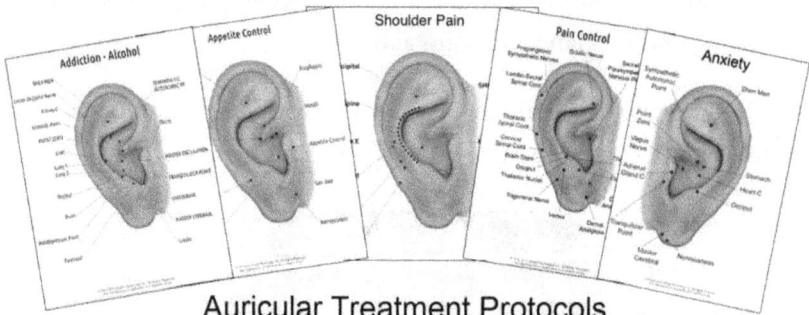

Auricular Treatment Protocols

ANALGESIC ANTIPHLOGISTIC ANTIPRURITIC

MYORELAXANT SKELETAL MUSCLES
ANXIOLYTIC ANTIDEPRESSANT ANTIALLERGIC

EATING DISORDERS

SUBSTANCE ADDICTIONS (TOBACCO AND ALCOHOL)

Advantages:

It is a relatively simple technique to apply, the points are in a limited and accessible area. The patient does not have to undress, it can be practiced on oneself and could also be used by "non-medical" figures; almost free of side effects or unwanted; effective on a wide range of pathologies, reduces or cancels the use of drugs, quick as application and as the appearance of results, finally also very inexpensive;

CHAPTER 22

EXAMPLES OF AURICULAR THERAPY

1) Auricular therapy for smoking cessation

2) Auricular therapy for dependencies

3) Auricular Acupuncture Weight Loss

4) Auricular therapy for headache

5) Auricular acupuncture points for lower back pain treatment.

7) Auricular therapy for insomnia and Stress

8) Auricular therapy for Allergies

9) Auricular therapy for toothache

10) Auricular therapy for depression

1) Auriculotherapy for smoking cessation

From-https://www.nobelpharm.com/smoking_cessation.html

Auricular therapy for smoking cessation was first used in the 1970's and has recently grown in popularity. It is a very effective approach with high success rates of about 80%. The secret is that auricular therapy stimulates a kind of natural chemical in the brain, called "endorphins". The endorphins bind to the specific neuro receptor, which nicotine used to fill. The body thinks it is "nicotine", so there's no withdrawal symptoms during non-smoking period. Without exposure to nicotine, the body slowly loses its addictiveness. The smokers no longer crave for smoking. Their psychological dependence is also broken. Quit smoking successfully!

Smoking Withdrawal

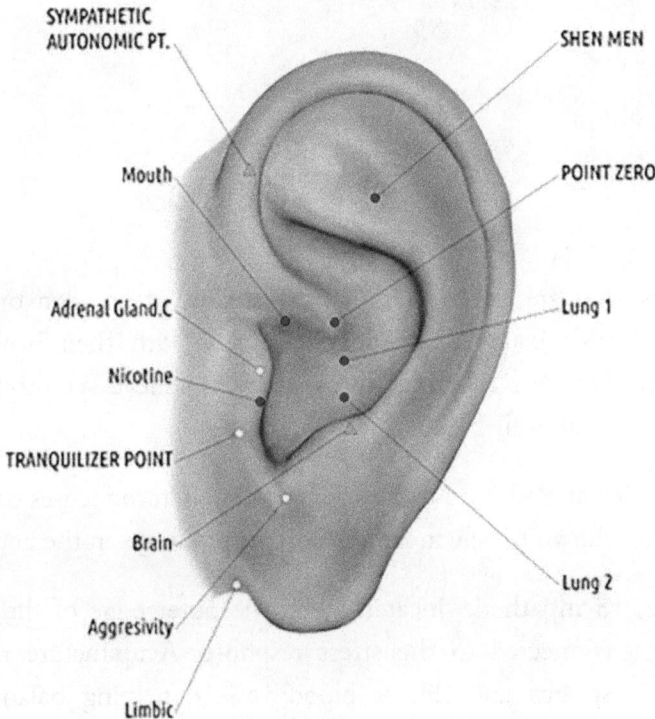

SYMPATHETIC AUTONOMIC PT.

SHEN MEN

Mouth

POINT ZERO

Adrenal Gland.C

Lung 1

Nicotine

TRANQUILIZER POINT

Brain

Lung 2

Aggresivity

Limbic

2) Auricular therapy for dependencies

From: https://www.beebehealthcare.org/health-hub/
conditions/listen-ear-acupuncture-resounds-promise-
managing-pain-anxiety-and-depression

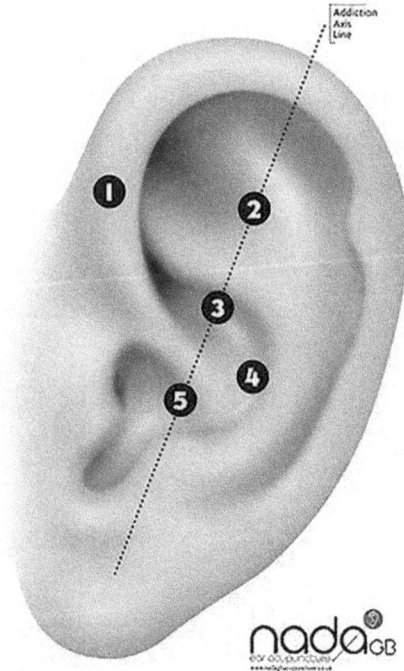

Patients who are experiencing severe anxiety, depression or other
mental health issues may want to consult with their healthcare
provider about ear acupuncture as a way to relieve symptoms and
improve overall well-being.

Five Auricular Pathways to Relief. Ear acupuncture focuses on these
five areas, shown to be connected to other pathways in the body:

1.   Sympathetic, located along the outer edge of the ear, is
     connected to the stress response. Acupuncture releases
     spasms and dilates blood vessels, helping balance the

autonomic nervous system, which controls breathing, the heartbeat and digestive processes.

2.   Shen Men, an oval-shaped depression inside the upper ear, is also known as the Spirit Gate. Acupuncture in this area is believed to anchor the spirit and calm the mind, used to help patients deal with insomnia, pain management, hyperactivity, high blood pressure, fear, and panic attacks.

3.   Kidney, in the ear's center, is known as the water element, and is at the root of Chinese medicine's yin and yang balance for optimal health. Acupuncture in this area, thought to control the essence of graceful aging, can help strengthen lower legs, spine and bone marrow, improve digestion and fertility and more. It is also used to help calm fear, paranoia and mistrust, and boost confidence.

4.   Liver, found along the ridge inside the ear, the wooden element is connected to regulating blood flow. Acupuncture provides relief for metabolic functions, such as nourishing the liver, ligaments, skin, nails and hair, and helping regulate menstruation, sleep, mood, and digestion. Stimulating this area with acupuncture is also helpful in dealing with emotions of anger, violence, frustration, or depression.

5.   Lung, the area on the lower side of the ear ridge, known as the metal element, controls respiration and functions of the skin. Acupuncture is associated with clearing up imbalances of apathy, lethargy, lack of inspiration, and grief

3) Auricular Acupuncture Weight Loss

From https://www.healthcmi.com/Acupuncture-Continuing-Education-News/1218-auricular-acupuncture-weight-loss-found-effective

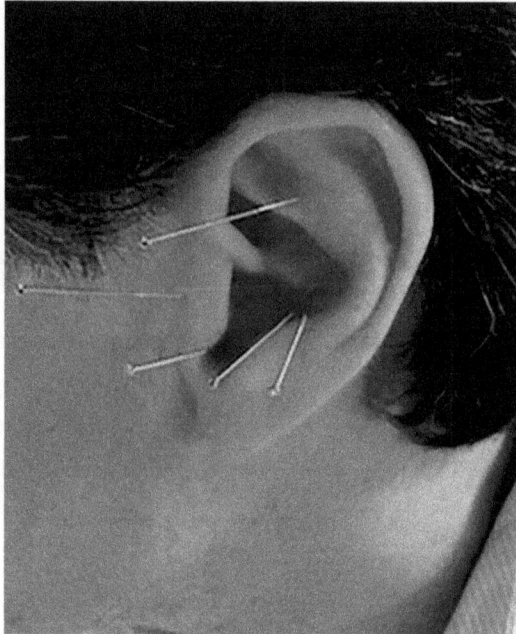

Auricular acupuncture successfully treats obesity. A new study concludes that a special 5 point combination of auricular acupuncture points is effective for weight loss in overweight individuals. Ear acupuncture for the treatment of obesity and hunger is depicted here.

Ear Acupuncture

A one-point auricular treatment was also found effective but not to the degree of clinical success as the 5 acupuncture point combination.

The five auricular acupuncture points: shenmen, spleen, stomach, hunger, endocrine.

4) Auricular therapy for headache

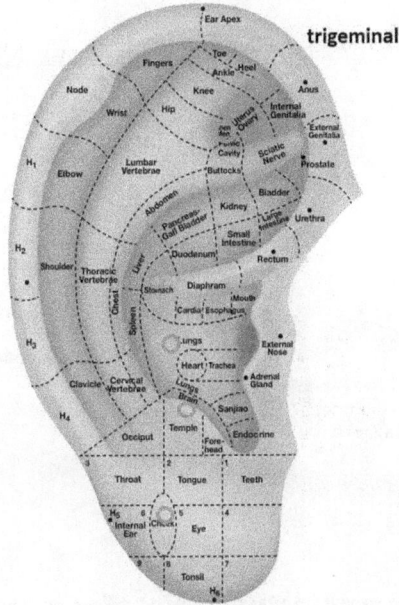

trigeminal

Headache - Migraine

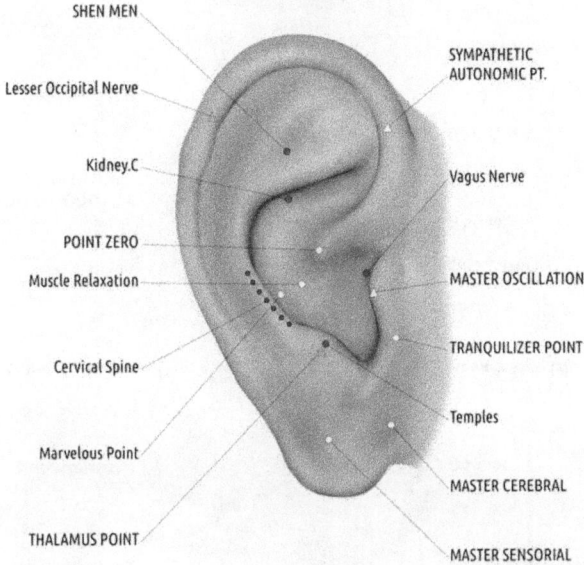

SHEN MEN

Lesser Occipital Nerve

Kidney.C

POINT ZERO

Muscle Relaxation

Cervical Spine

Marvelous Point

THALAMUS POINT

SYMPATHETIC AUTONOMIC PT.

Vagus Nerve

MASTER OSCILLATION

TRANQUILIZER POINT

Temples

MASTER CEREBRAL

MASTER SENSORIAL

5) Auricular acupuncture points for lower back pain treatment.

From: https://www.hindawi.com/journals/ecam/2012/383257/

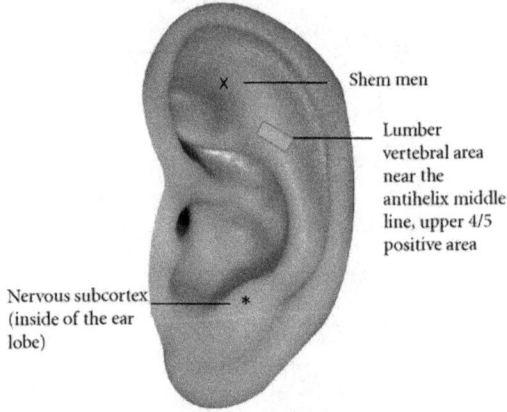

Shem men

Lumber vertebral area near the antihelix middle line, upper 4/5 positive area

Nervous subcortex (inside of the ear lobe)

6) Auricular acupuncture points for hypertension

Hypertension

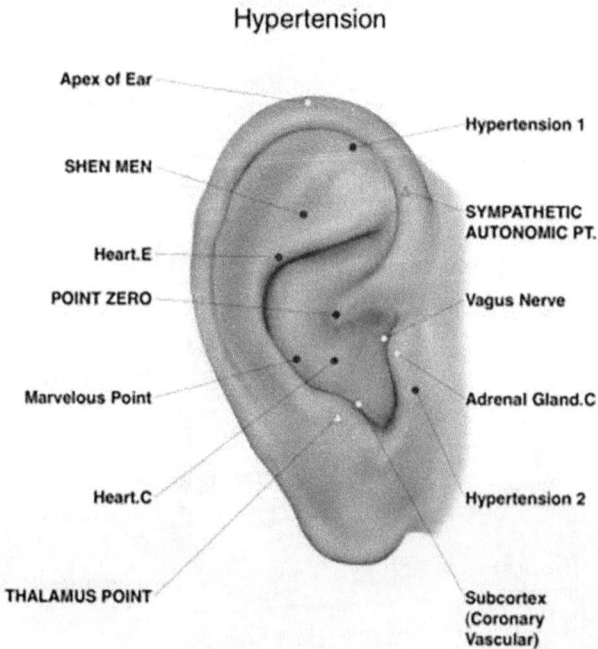

Apex of Ear

Hypertension 1

SHEN MEN

SYMPATHETIC AUTONOMIC PT.

Heart.E

POINT ZERO

Vagus Nerve

Marvelous Point

Adrenal Gland.C

Heart.C

Hypertension 2

THALAMUS POINT

Subcortex (Coronary Vascular)

7) Auricular therapy for insomnia and stress

Ear Reflexology For Insomnia & Better Sleep

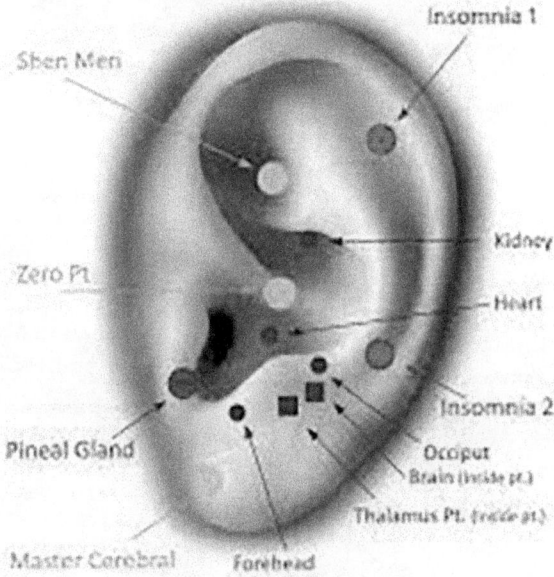

Shen Men

Insomnia 1

Zero Pt

Kidney

Heart

Pineal Gland

Insomnia 2

Occiput
Brain (inside pt.)

Thalamus Pt. (inside pt.)

Master Cerebral

Forehead

Color Points are Primary Points. Blue Points are secondary points.

http://www.goodnurture.com/2012/01/reflexology-
for-insomnia-and-better.html?m=1.

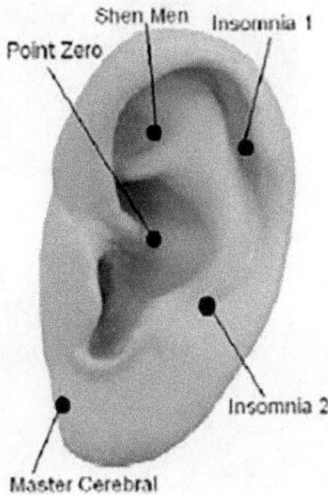

Shen Men

Insomnia 1

Point Zero

Insomnia 2

Master Cerebral

153

Stress

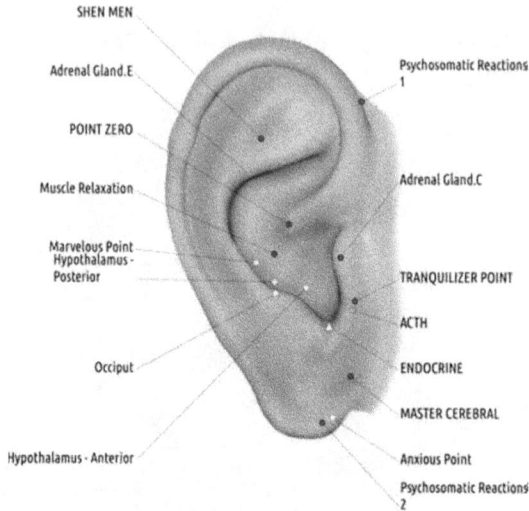

SHEN MEN

Adrenal Gland.E

POINT ZERO

Muscle Relaxation

Marvelous Point
Hypothalamus -
Posterior

Occiput

Hypothalamus - Anterior

Psychosomatic Reactions
1

Adrenal Gland.C

TRANQUILIZER POINT

ACTH

ENDOCRINE

MASTER CEREBRAL

Anxious Point

Psychosomatic Reactions
2

8) Auricular therapy for Allergies

allergie

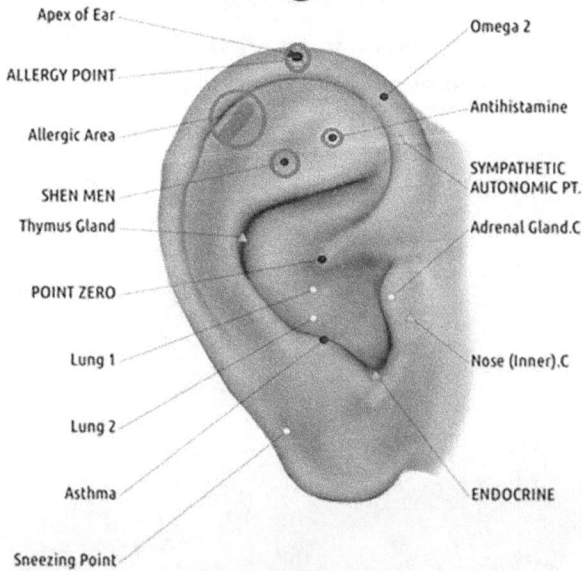

Apex of Ear

ALLERGY POINT

Allergic Area

SHEN MEN

Thymus Gland

POINT ZERO

Lung 1

Lung 2

Asthma

Sneezing Point

Omega 2

Antihistamine

SYMPATHETIC
AUTONOMIC PT.

Adrenal Gland.C

Nose (Inner).C

ENDOCRINE

Allergy

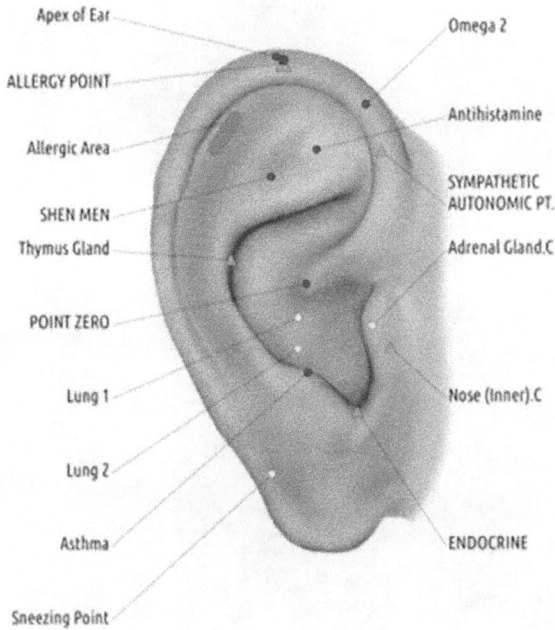

Apex of Ear

ALLERGY POINT

Allergic Area

SHEN MEN

Thymus Gland

POINT ZERO

Lung 1

Lung 2

Asthma

Sneezing Point

Omega 2

Antihistamine

SYMPATHETIC AUTONOMIC PT.

Adrenal Gland.C

Nose (Inner).C

ENDOCRINE

© 2010-2012 Miridia Technology Inc., All Rights Reserved
Any reproduction or duplication is a violation of law

9) Auricular therapy for toothache

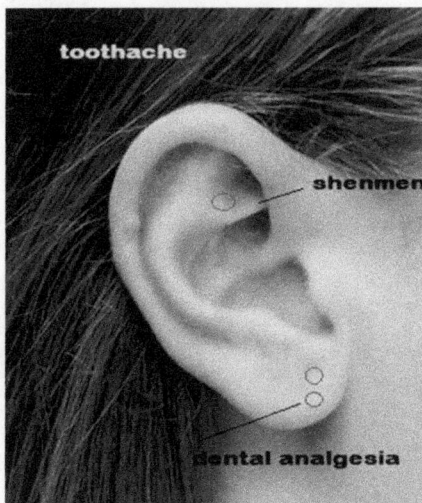

toothache

shenmen

dental analgesia

155

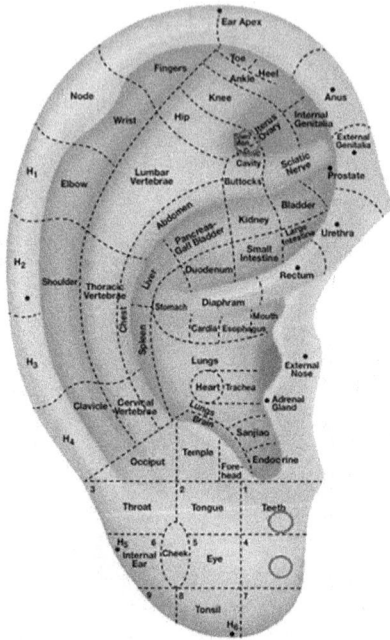

10) Auricular therapy for depression

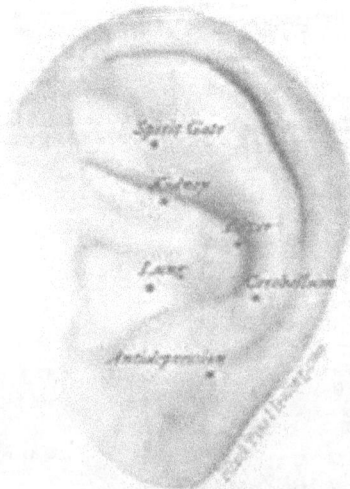

Depression

AURICULAR ACUPUNCTURE

BOX 3.5

MAIN EAR POINTS FOR DEPRESSION

1. **Sympathetic**
   - at the medial end of the
     of the inferior crus of the
     antihelix, where the crus
     of the helix and antihelix
     intersect (also known as
     Autonomic point)

2. **Anti-depression**
   - on the ear lobe, at the
     intersection of a line running
     from the lower edge of the
     intertragic notch and the
     postantitragal fossa (AKA
     cheerfulness point)

3. **Shenmen**
   - slightly above the angle
     formed by the superior and
     inferior antihelical crura

4. **Zero point**
   - on the ascending crus of the
     helix as it starts to rise from
     the superior concha, in a
     small yet distinct fossa

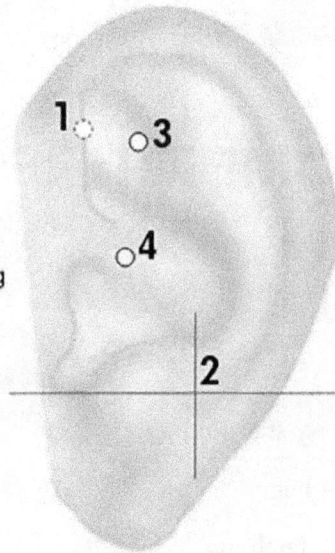

◌ *Dotted line indicates
a point inside the ear.*

CHAPTER 23

SOME INTERESTING POINTS

12 sky star points
....

Li 4 hegu
....

Lv 3 taichong
....

Li 11 qu chi
....

There are just over thirty acupuncture points that are most important and which are mostly used. In practice those that are used for the most common discomforts are a little less.

In the previous chapters we have already seen some points for treating, namely

- ➲ back pain
- ➲ the frozen shoulder
- ➲ sleeping and eating disorders
- ➲ dampness

Let us now look at a group of interesting points. A famous Taoist physician and monk, Ma Dan Yang (1123 - 1183) lived during the Song Dynasty. composed an ode celebrating and describing the wonders of 11 miraculous points that could heal all diseases. These points were located along the meridians of the 'intestines, lung, heart, stomach, biliary and urinary bladder. This sonnet is considered a starting point for the study of acupuncture and moxibustion. In harmony with the brightest stars in the sky, it is said, they melted pains like warm water on snow. In 1329 another great master, Xu Feng, collected this data and had it published in the Jade Dragon Manual under the name of the 12 star points of the sky, with the addition of Lv 3, a very important point, on the liver meridian, is not to be forgotten.

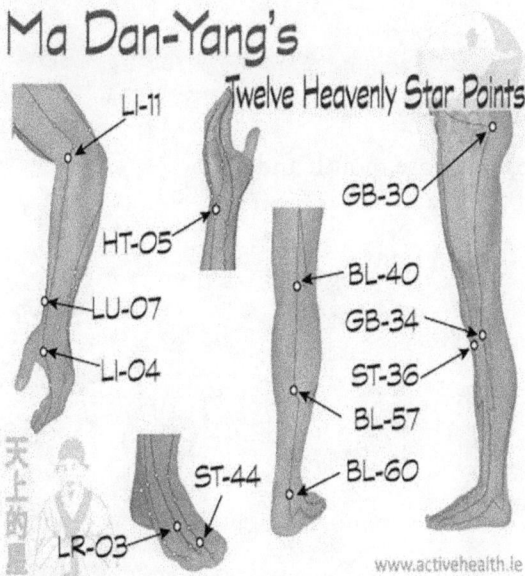

Ma Dan-Yang's Twelve Heavenly Star Points

LI-11
HT-05
LU-07
LI-04
LR-03
ST-44
GB-30
BL-40
GB-34
ST-36
BL-57
BL-60

www.activehealth.ie

These are the famous twelve points of the star in the sky.

**Li 4, Lv 3, Li 11, Lu 7, Ht 5, Bl 40, Bl 57,
Bl 60, Gb 30, Gb 34, St 36, St 44**

Let us look at some of them in detail

Li 4 hegu (meeting in the valley).

Most commonly used point ever.

It is easy to find and easy to deal with. It comes in combination with many other points, especially Lv 3 of the foot. Same position with respect to the first two toes.

The combination of these 4 points are called the 4 gates of pain. Historically this faculty is reported to reduce all pains in the whole body. The point on the hand, Li 4, is thought to affect pains in the upper part of the body, while Lv 3 in the lower part.

Actions:

regulates sweating
expels wind
regulates face, eyes,nose,mouth and ears
relieves pain

MODERN REFLEXOLOGY

LI 4

RELIEVES:

* A headache
* Eye problems
* Skin diseases
* Fever
* Boosts the immune system

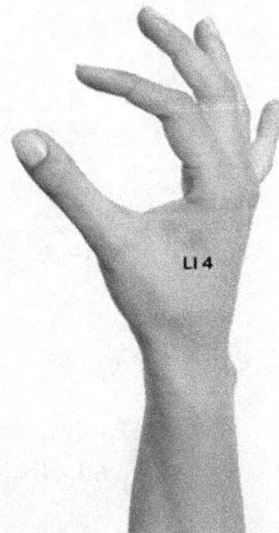

LI 4

Contra Indicated during Pregnancy Joining Valley

He Gu LI-04

Indications:

Dispels, exterior Wind, Releases the Exterior, Stimulates the dispersing function of the Lungs, Stops pain, Removes obstructions from channel by activating the channel and alleviates pain, Tonifies Qi and consolidates the Exterior, Harmonises ascending and descending, Regulates the defensive Qi and adjusts sweating, Regulates the face, eyes, nose, mouth and ears, Induces labour, Restores the Yang.

Location:

Midway between the junction of the 1st. and 2nd metacarpal bones (fingers) and the margin of the web.

www.activehealth.ie

Lv 3 Chinese name: Tai Chong
English name: Great Rushing

It is the second most important point and the most widely used. Indicated for all lower body pain, combined with Li 4 it forms the four gates of pain. It has an infinite number of applications and almost always enters all therapeutic protocols. To name a few: hypertension, allergies, insomnia , depression, regulates menstruation, strengthens the immune system and promotes general rebalancing.

Acupuncture Point
LV3 (Taichong)

- Spreads Liver Qi
- Nourishes Liver blood and Liver yin
- Regulates menstruation
- Regulates the lower jiao

MODERN REFLEXOLOGY

▌ LI 11 Qu Chi

Actions:

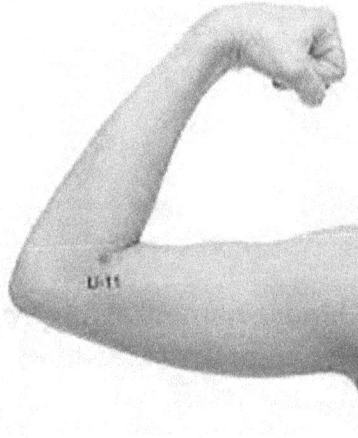

purifies heat
cools the blood
eliminates wind
drains moisture and relieves itching

Indications:

fever
painful throat obstruction
loss of voice
agitation
manic syndrome
upper limb tingling and skin diseases

CHAPTER 24

OTHER POINTS OF THE FOOT

K 1, YONGQUAN gushing spring

Shimian

Taixi KI-3 Great Stream

Zhaohai k 6 High seas

Bl 60 kun lun

A s a podiatrist, I have studied deeply the many wonders of the foot, its convolutions with various health problems, I could not help but mention some of its interesting points .

I would like to highlight five points, in addition to the aforementioned and famous Liver 3 in the previous chapter.

Two points of some significance are found on the plant. The first is

K 1, YONGQUAN gushing spring,

Which is the first point of the Kidney meridian.

The second point, Shimian, somewhat less famous than the first, being an off-meridian point, is located in the center of the heel and is called the point of insomnia because of its recognized relaxing properties.

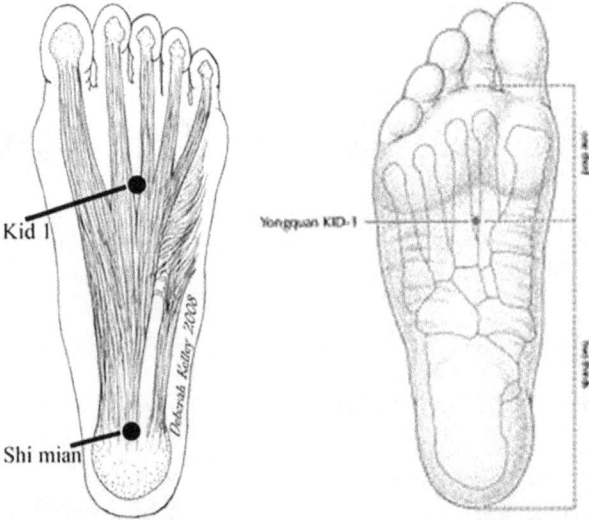

Let's look at this special point in more detail

location: between the second and third metatarsal bones

actions:

brings down the 'excess from the head
sedates the wind
calms the shen
restores consciousness
restores yang

indications:

loss of consciousness
epilepsy
hypertension
agitation
insomnia
sexual problems
pain in the feet

Indications:

For weak feet and knees, poor memory, impotence, low back pain, warm sensation in the soles of the feet, sleep disturbances, pain in the soles of the feet, dizziness, vertex headaches, nosebleeds, visual disturbances, irritability, calf cramps, neck and back pain, throat swelling, fever, syncope, shock, fatigue, adinamia, constipation or diarrhea, gastralgias, tightness in the chest, asthma, jaundice, urination disorders, cough, thirst, "internal heat" diseases, heat stroke, apoplexy, hypertonia, epilepsy, toothache. Roots man to the earth.

Very useful for childhood convulsions (jing) and epilepsy (xian).

Best technique: massage and moxibustion

According to the Chinese, the main actions are: calming shen, eliminating heat and fire, lowering excessive yang , calming wind and restoring consciousness and willpower. It is used in excess conditions when the upper body is involved especially.

The name gushing (bubbling) spring renders well the idea of energy, and vitality taking strength from the earth. Another name is: Source of Life . This is, in fact, the only point on the sole of the foot (according to classical acupuncture) and the lowest point of the body therefore closest to the earth.

The kidneys belong to 'water and this to the feeling of fear.

This point is not much used in acupuncture because it is painful, however it is one of the most famous and well-known points both treated manually with pressure and with moxa. Some naturopaths suggest stepping on a tennis ball to stimulate the sole of the foot, starting right at Yonquan.

Manual stimulation of this point can provide interesting insights into a person's level of nerve tension. Normally when a lot of pressure is applied, you get a very noticeable type of reaction, like an electric shock, especially in people who are very sensitive to stress, or otherwise have a high level of cortisol.

I remember that cortisol is a stress-related hormone and it is activated, just by the adrenal glands, which are located above the kidneys.

It is thought , in fact, that this kind of manipulation can significantly lower its level. So you can use this point, before going to bed to promote general relaxation and better sleep quality.

By using moxa at this point you get a good dose of energy that is transferred throughout the body. It is said that in Korea, in ancient times, there was a tradition that recommended that young bachelors

166

before getting married walk on hot coals for at least a month to enhance their sexual activity.

Comment: related to fear and anxiety, much used in massage, little in acupuncture because very painful

Combinations with other points for other therapies

anti-aging: K 1, Sp 6, St 36, Li 4, Tb 23

For insomnia: Pc 6, Sp 6, Ht 7, K 6, Bl 62, Du 20, St 36, K 1.

Headaches and dizziness: K 1, St 2, Bl 11

Loss of voice K 1, Li 4, Gb 35

Intense thirst K 1, Lv 2

Menopausal hot flashes K 1, Lv 3, Ht 6, ren 4

Stiffness and lower back pain: K 1, Du 2, Bl 40, Bl 27, Bl 28

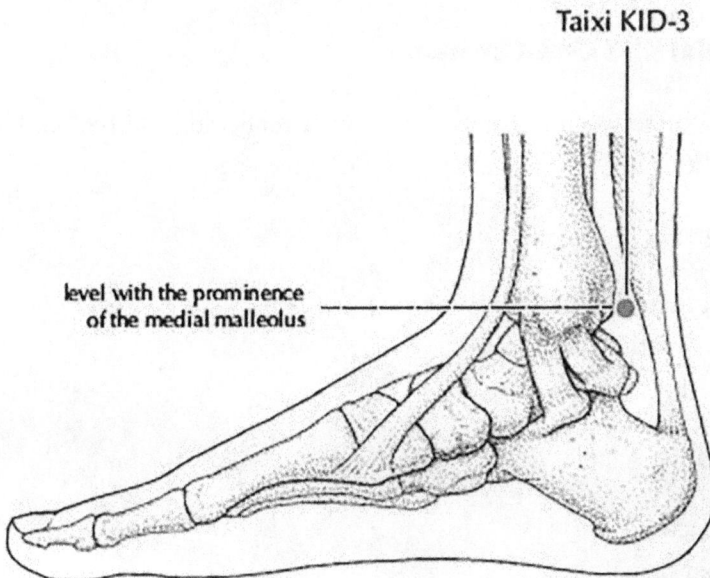

Taixi KID-3

level with the prominence of the medial malleolus

Traditional Chinese Medicine

Tai Xi — KI-03

Strengthen the Kidneys
Benefits Essence
Nourishes Kidney Yin
Cools empty Heat
Cultivate Kidney Yang
Strengthens the lower back and knees
Anchors the Qi and benefits the Lung
Harmonise the uterus

Location: In the depression between the medial malleolus and the tendo calcaneus, at the level with the tip of the medial malleolus.

online course at www.activehealth.ie

https://nl.pinterest.com/pin/340725528028516799/

Taixi KI-3 Great Stream

location: between the apex of the inner malleolus and the tendon of Achilles.

actions:

strengthens the lumbar spine
nourishes the kidney Yin
tones the Yang kidney

indications:

toothache
lumbar pains

agitation

insomnia

sexual and urogenital problems

increases fertility

pain in the soles of the feet

Very important point to tone the deficient kidney for any reason.

"Current Supreme" is another name by which this point became famous. It's an important point of toning, because it acts on the Yin and Yang of the kidney. It's used to treat many chronic disorders. In particular toothache , insomnia, excessive dreamlike activity, poor memory, impotence, seminal emission, premature ejaculation, sexual exhaustion, irregular menstruation, low back pain. Cold in the lower limbs, numbness and pain in the legs, swelling and pain in the ankles and heel.

Taixi KI-3 has long been used to treat empty kidney lumbar pain and is also indicated for kidney heel pain, traumatic damage or painful obstruction. When treating the heel, the point should be manipulated until you get a feeling that radiates strongly downwards.

A widely used technique for ankle pain is to simultaneously press the BL-60 Kunlun point on the opposite side with the thumb and the index finger.

Combinations with other points.

Kidney Empty Lumbar Pain: K 3, Bl 23, Bl 40, Bl 30

Ankle pain: K 3, Bl 60

Pain in the penis: K 3, Lu 10, Ren 3

Hypertension K 3, Sp 6, Lv 3, Gb 39, Bl 60, Cv 4, Lu 9

Zhaohai k 6 High Seas

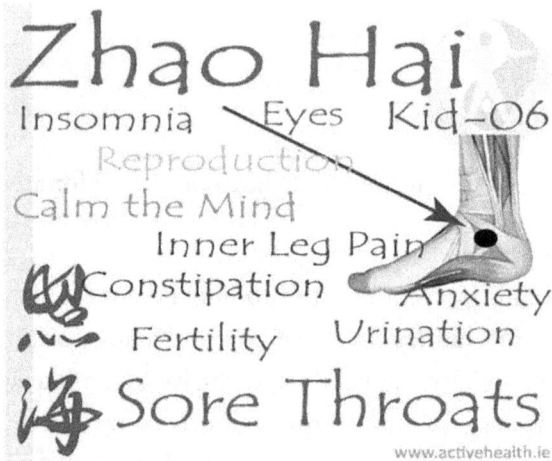

Zhao Hai
Insomnia   Eyes   Kid–O6
Reproduction
Calm the Mind
        Inner Leg Pain
Constipation   Anxiety
    Fertility   Urination
Sore Throats
www.activehealth.ie

location: under the prominence of the medial malleolus

actions:

nourish and humidify the Yin,
refresh the body, eliminate the empty heat
calms the shen

indications:

swelling of the throat
eye pain, disturbed vision dizziness
agitation , insomnia
gynecological disorders
genital itching

comment: excellent results with moxa and massage. Used to restore communication and balance between heart and kidneys, water and fire.

Action:

It stimulates the rise of renal Qi, regulates the Lungs, the Heart and the Liver, purifies the Heat, calms the Shen.

Indications:

Dryness of the throat, depression, melancholy, fatigue, feeling of heaviness in the limbs, insomnia, inappetence, cold hands and feet, pain, abdominal "masses", urination disorders, poor urine, polyuria, tendency to wince, fever, night seizures, menstrual disorders, vulval itching, prolapse of the uterus, leucorrhea, pain in the eyes, spasms in the throat, laryngitis, ataxia, cerebellar disorders, disorders of walking.

Combinations with other points

For insomnia: Pc 6, Sp 6, Ht 7, K 6, Bl 62, Du 20, St 36, K 1.

Bl 60 kun lun

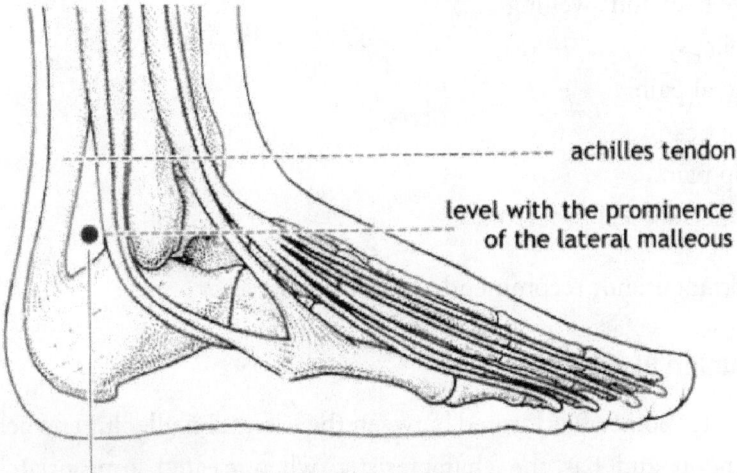

achilles tendon

level with the prominence of the lateral malleous

Kunlun BL-60   Source: A Manual of Acupuncture

Other names:

Fire Point
Point of Late Summer
Jing or River Point
Heavenly Star Point
Aspirin point

location: between the lateral malleolus and the Achilles tendon

actions:

Facilitates the circulation of Qi of the channel
relaxes the tendons and strengthens the lumbar spine
induces childbirth
relieves the pain
eliminates the heat in the head

indications:

eye pain and swelling
epilepsy
sacral pain
sciatica
hip pain
gynecological problems

comment: not recommended during pregnancy

Kunlun BL-60 mountains

Blister point 60 is located between the external malleolus and achilles tendon and has the characteristic, when treated appropriately, of relieving various pains. The main indications are: headache, nuchal stiffness, dizziness, shoulder and back cramps, spasms and paresis of the limbs, infantile seizures and tics, swelling of the ankles and knees, foot pain, swelling of the genital organs, and difficult childbirth. It is considered the **aspirin point**, useful for almost any pain, and as evidenced by the many traditional accounts it is one of the most important points for relieving back tension. Some say that the discovery, just, of this point ignited that much curiosity that sparked subsequent studies of acupuncture points.

It is said, that a few thousand years ago, in China, during a hunting trip in the mountains a hunter saw something like the fur of a small animal under the snow and shot an arrow that hit the mark. But to his amazement he discovered that it was not an animal but the peculiar footwear worn by a colleague who had fallen asleep , under the snow. The victim, struck at the point between malleolus and tendon naturally woke up in pain but was then so happy to find that all the pain he had been complaining of in his back for years had miraculously disappeared.

Proponents of moxa, who claim that this technique even predates acupuncture tell another story instead. At the end of a stop around the fire , some soldiers, began to tidy up their things to leave again and one of them took it upon himself to 'put out the fire. So it was that the poor soldier began, in haste, to step on the ashes and burning embers and ended up getting burned around an ankle. As is often the case, it is spontaneous to vigorously massage the sore spot to relieve the pain. Here, too, the pain of the burn was offset by the disappearance of all the aches and pains from which he had long suffered.

From American Dragon:

'This is an important point to clear Excess Wind, Fire and Yang from the upper part of the body.

This is a key point for testing heroine and cocaine addiction, it will be tender.

Kunlun is a mountain range near tibet. It is also a name for Mount Everest and a name for Chinese Paradise - the source of enlightenment.

This point stimulates the pituitary gland and the testes.

When using this point, you are contacting the persons Spirit with the essence and quality of Fire and warming it.

This point is better for chronic rather than acute back pain and better for Deficiency than Excess.

One source says to use UB-60 Kunlun for the upper back and UB-40 Weizhong for the lower back. '

CHAPTER 25

POSSIBLE REMEDIES

Some suggestions for possible remedies offered by integrative medicine (acupuncture,digito pressure, massage, moxibustion) for The most common ailments.

Weight control
....

Hypertension
....

Headaches
....

Back pain
....

Insomnia and stress
....

Depression
....

Allergies
....

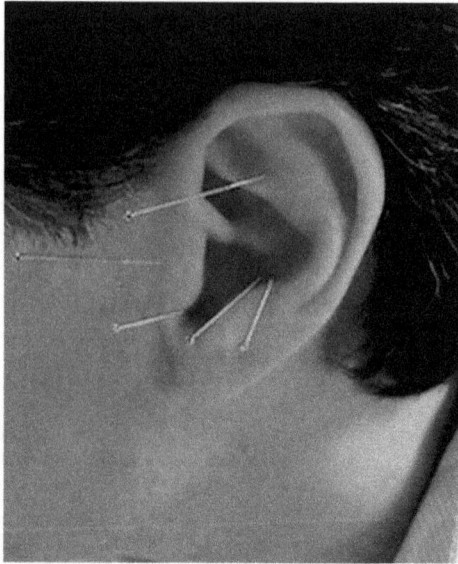

weight control

Some integrated treatment suggestions

Ear points: Shen men, hunger point , stomach spleen, endocrine

Obesity or difficulty in succeeding in maintaining optimal weight can have several underlying causes.

Acupressure/acupuncture

(a) Heat in the Stomach Stasis of heat and moisture:
Zusanli ST 36 Neiting ST 44 Fenglong ST 40
Sanyinjiao SP 6 Hegu LI 4 Quchi LI 11

(b) Spleen deficiency and moisture stagnation:
Pishu BL 20 Weishu BL 21 Sanyinjiao SP 6
Zusanli ST 36 Fenglong ST 40

c) Kidney deficiency:
Pishu BL 20 Shensh BL 23 Sanyinjiao SP 6
Mingmen GV 4 Taixi KI 3

Reduce stress: with breathing and relaxation exercises, Qi cong, yoga, regular physical activity

Dietary suggestions: drink a lot, (green tea, decoctions and hunger-breaking herbal teas made from mallow leaves, lemon balm, passion flower, ash, ginger) a lot of fruits and vegetables. Choose low-glycemic index, low-calorie, alkalizing, antioxidant foods. Limit dinner to only vegetables and vegetable protein.

HYPERTENSION:

6 points on the foot: Ki 3, Sp 6, Lv 3, St 41, Gb 39, Bl 60

6 points on the body: Pc 6, St 36, Li 4, Gb 20, Gv 20, Li 11

4 points on the hear: Shen men, Point Zero, Hypertension1, 2

Hypertension

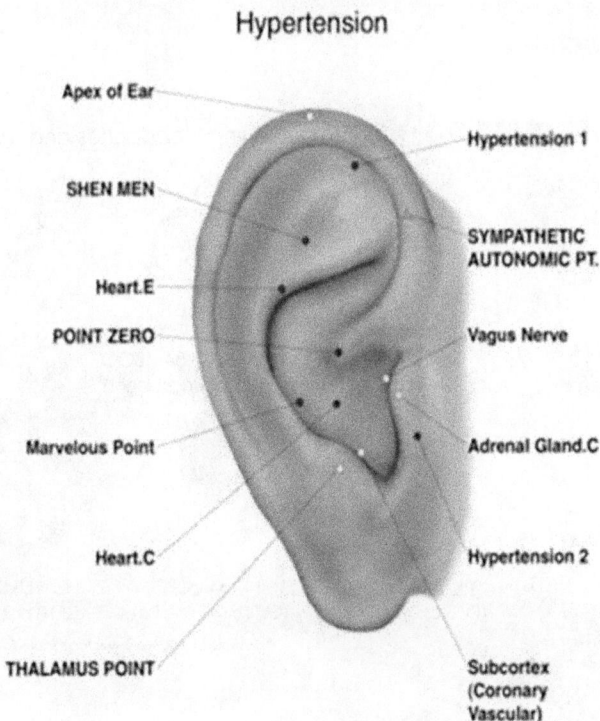

177

Hypertension

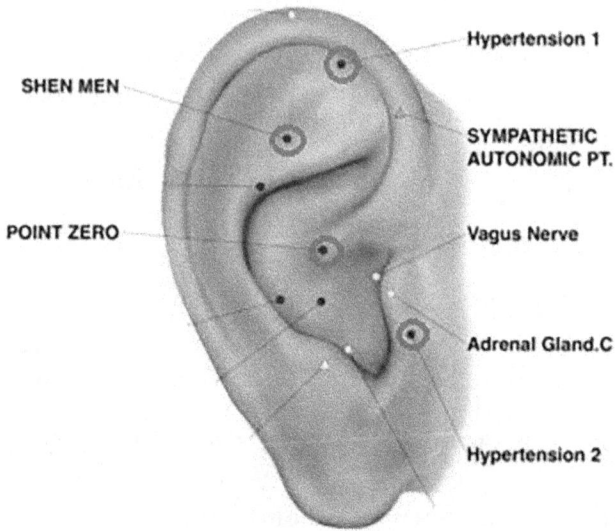

- Hypertension 1
- SHEN MEN
- SYMPATHETIC AUTONOMIC PT.
- POINT ZERO
- Vagus Nerve
- Adrenal Gland.C
- Hypertension 2

Headaches

ACUPRESSURE POINTS for Relieving Headaches and Migraines

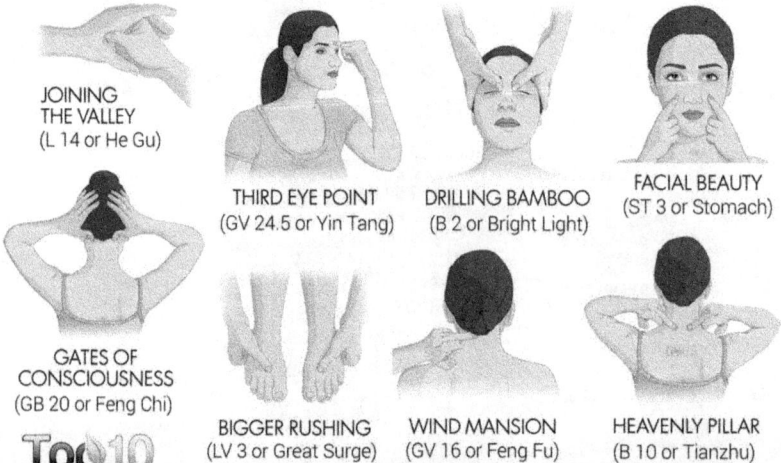

JOINING THE VALLEY
(L 14 or He Gu)

THIRD EYE POINT
(GV 24.5 or Yin Tang)

DRILLING BAMBOO
(B 2 or Bright Light)

FACIAL BEAUTY
(ST 3 or Stomach)

GATES OF CONSCIOUSNESS
(GB 20 or Feng Chi)

BIGGER RUSHING
(LV 3 or Great Surge)

WIND MANSION
(GV 16 or Feng Fu)

HEAVENLY PILLAR
(B 10 or Tianzhu)

Top10 Home Remedies

To explore more, visit www.Top10HomeRemedies.com

Headache - Migraine

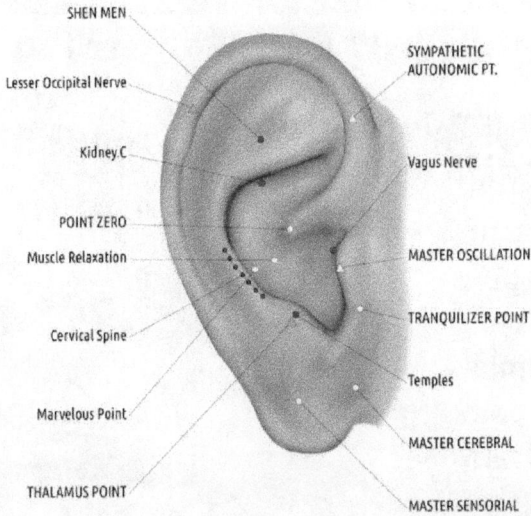

SHEN MEN

Lesser Occipital Nerve

Kidney.C

POINT ZERO

Muscle Relaxation

Cervical Spine

Marvelous Point

THALAMUS POINT

SYMPATHETIC AUTONOMIC PT.

Vagus Nerve

MASTER OSCILLATION

TRANQUILIZER POINT

Temples

MASTER CEREBRAL

MASTER SENSORIAL

Insomnia and stress

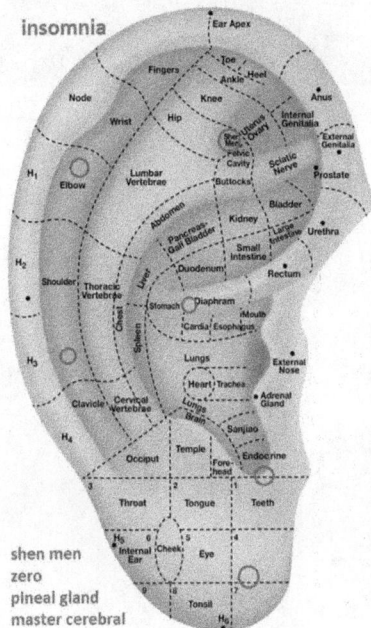

insomnia

shen men
zero
pineal gland
master cerebral

179

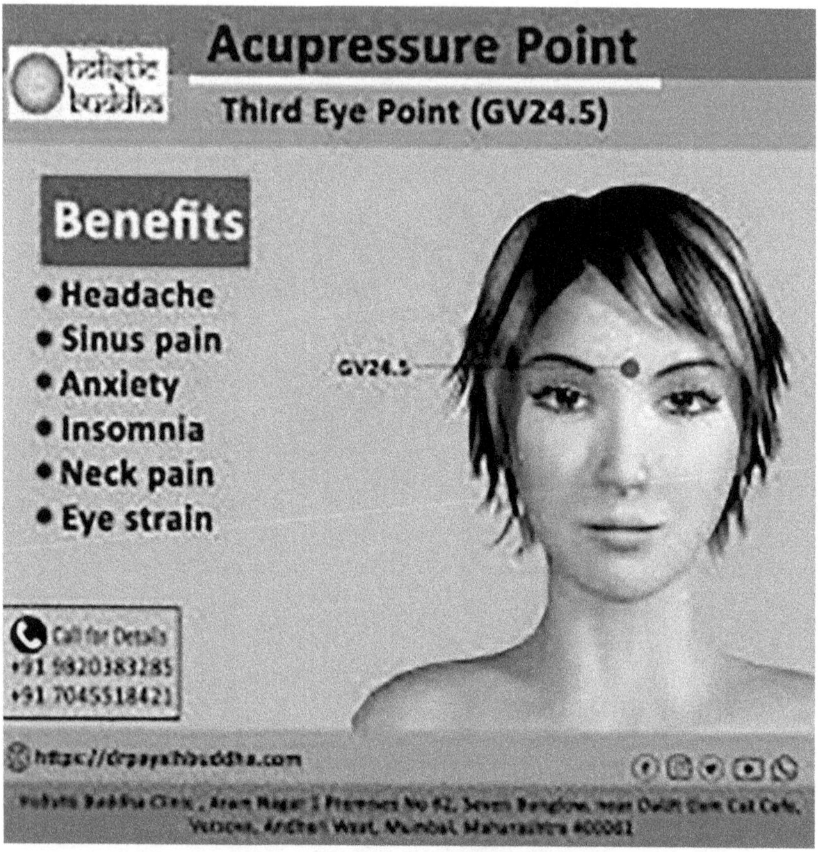
Acupressure Point
Third Eye Point (GV24.5)
Benefits
• Headache
• Sinus pain
• Anxiety
• Insomnia
• Neck pain
• Eye strain
GV24.5
Call for Details

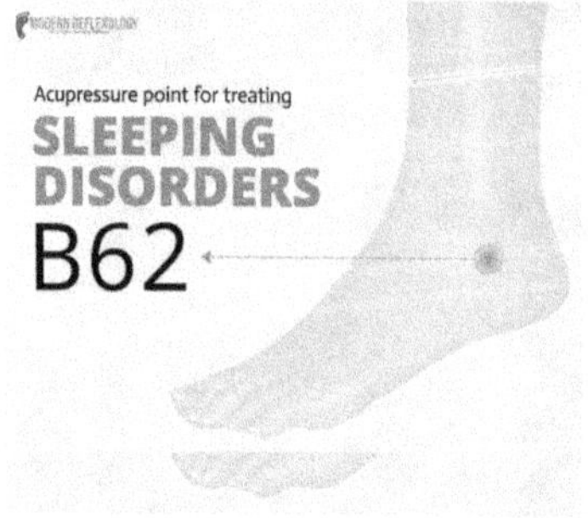
Acupressure point for treating
SLEEPING DISORDERS
B62

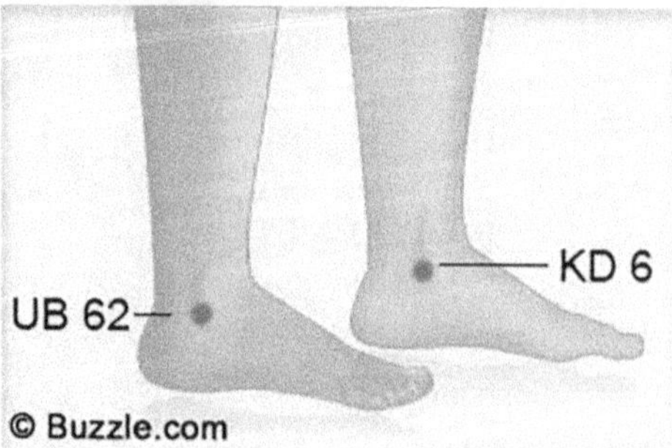
KD 6
UB 62
© Buzzle.com

Acupressure Treatment for Insomnia

Here are some best acupressure points that can be stimulated to relieve insomnia;
PC6, SP6, HT7, KD6, BL62, DU20, ST36, and KD1.

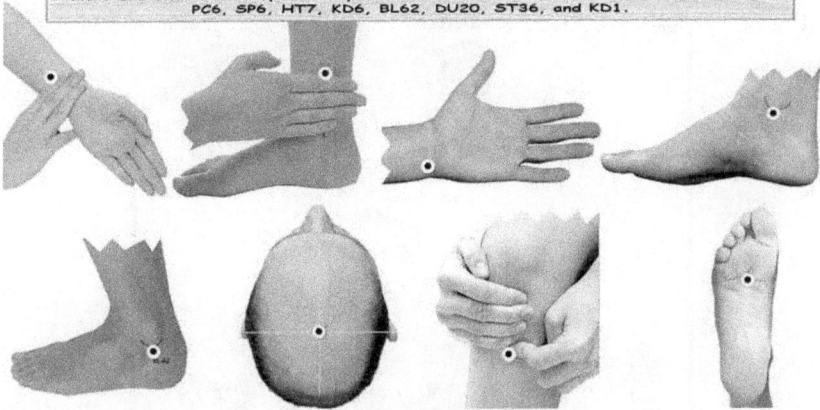

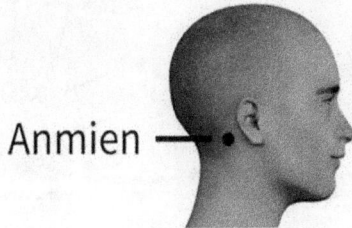

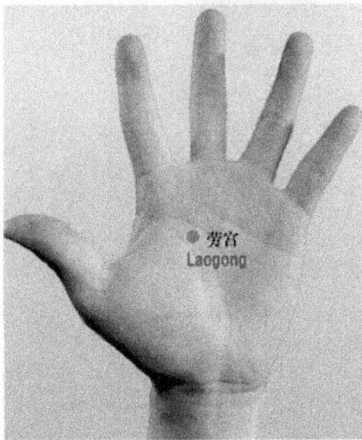

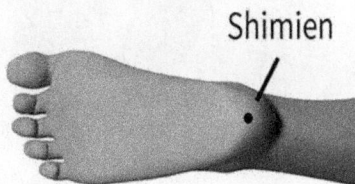

Anmien

● 劳宫
Laogong

Shimien

ACUPRESSURE POINTS TO TREAT BACKACHES

LOWER BACK POINTS
(Sea of Vitality)

STOMACH POINT
(Sea of Energy)

HIP BONE POINTS
(Womb & Vitals)

ELBOW POINT
(Cubit Marsh)

HAND POINT

KNEE POINTS
(Commanding Middle)

FOOT POINTS

Top10 Home Remedies   To explore more, visit www.Top10HomeRemedies.com

Back Pain - Low Back

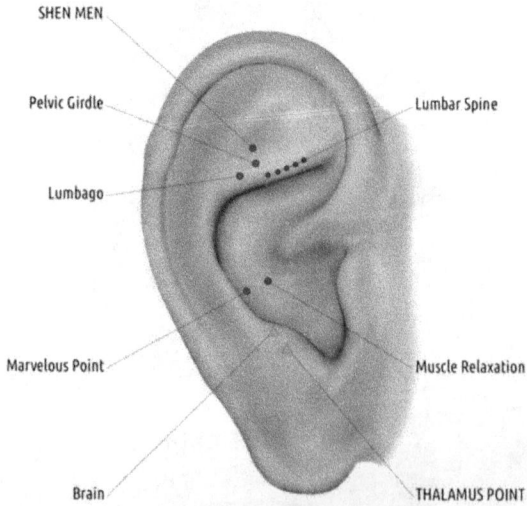

SHEN MEN

Pelvic Girdle

Lumbar Spine

Lumbago

Marvelous Point

Muscle Relaxation

Brain

THALAMUS POINT

Powerful Acupressure Points for Relieving Lower Back Pain

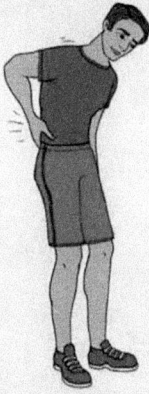

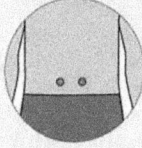
(BL 23)

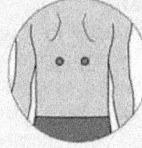
(BL 47)

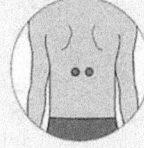
(GB 31)

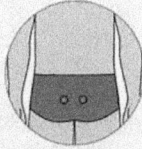
(GB 54)

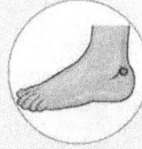
(BL 60)

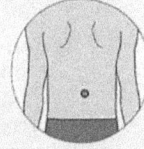
(GV 4)

MODERN REFLEXOLOGY

FIGHTS DEPRESSION

Press the point at the
center of the big toe
for a few minutes
2 or 3 times a day
to relieve depression
& anxiety.

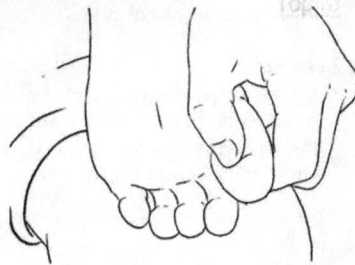

Top10
Home Remedies

BOX 3.5

MAIN EAR POINTS FOR DEPRESSION

1. Sympathetic
- at the medial end of the of the inferior crus of the antihelix, where the crus of the helix and antihelix intersect (also known as Autonomic point)

2. Anti-depression
- on the ear lobe, at the intersection of a line running from the lower edge of the intertragic notch and the postantitragal fossa (AKA cheerfulness point)

3. Shenmen
- slightly above the angle formed by the superior and inferior antihelical crura

4. Zero point
- on the ascending crus of the helix as it starts to rise from the superior concha, in a small yet distinct fossa

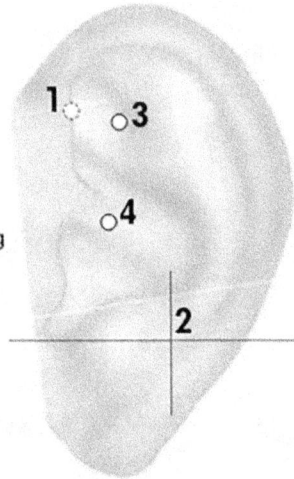

Dotted line indicates a point inside the ear.

Depression
AURICULAR ACUPUNCTURE

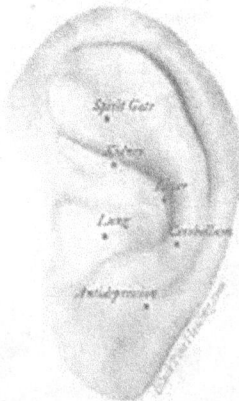

Spirit Gate

Lung

Antidepression

Allergies

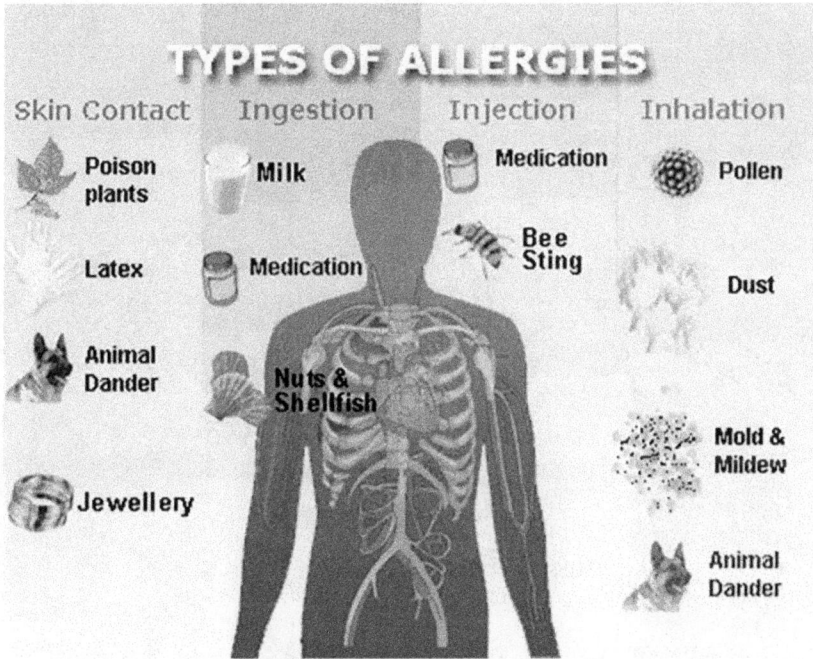

TYPES OF ALLERGIES

Skin Contact — Poison plants, Latex, Animal Dander, Jewellery

Ingestion — Milk, Medication, Nuts & Shellfish

Injection — Medication, Bee Sting

Inhalation — Pollen, Dust, Mold & Mildew, Animal Dander

https://fastreliefacupuncture.com/saat-allergy-treatments/

Allergies can also be caused by various factors. I suggest some possible remedies by stimulating points on the body and on the ear.

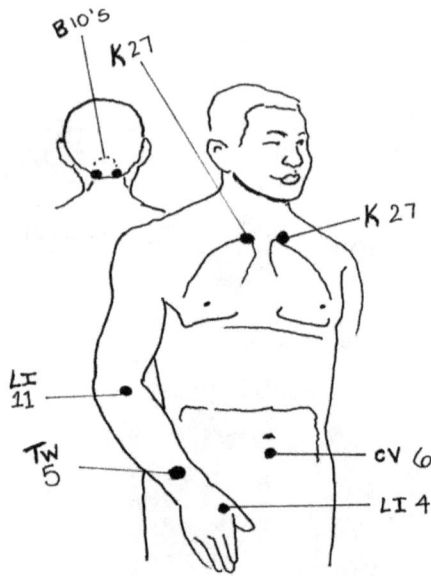

allergie

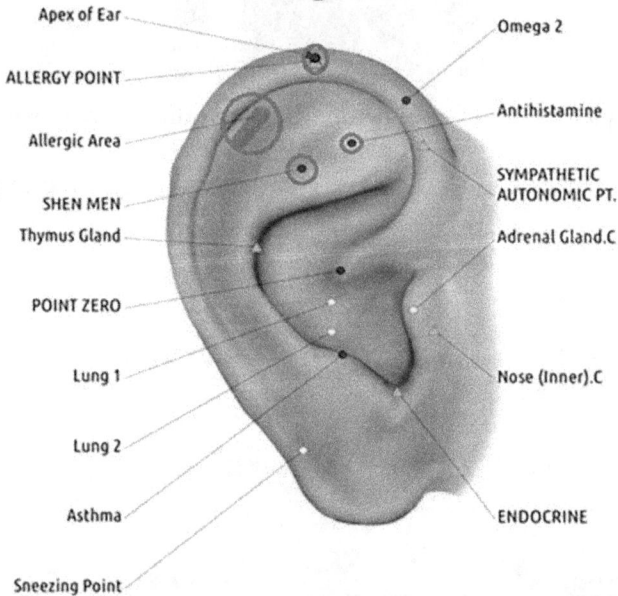

**Allerghttps://www.suburnett.com/
allergy-acupressure-points-for-us-humans/ies**

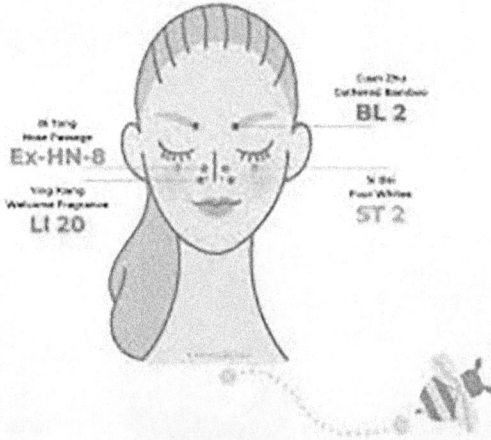

LOCAL ACUPOINTS FOR
SEASONAL ALLERGIES

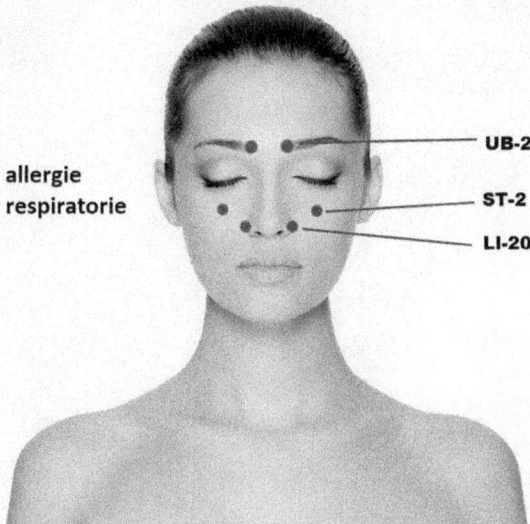

allergie
respiratorie

UB-2

ST-2

LI-20

https://fastreliefacupuncture.com/saat-allergy-treatments/

FINAL GREETING

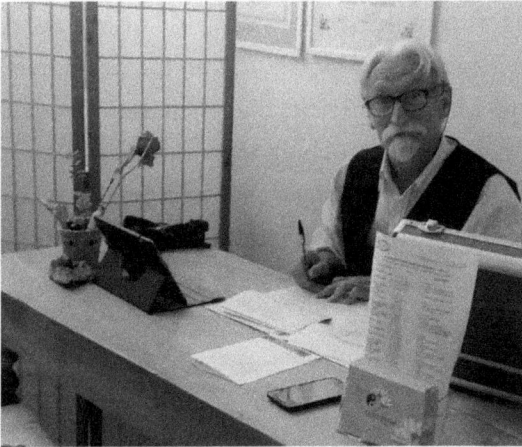

I hope that this kind of manual can be useful in some way to cope with some minor disturbance, perhaps not otherwise solvable by classical systems. An alternative or rather a supplement can always be convenient. For the more curious, I hope I have given an idea of how health problems are complex and that nevertheless there are many, sometimes, unthinkable solutions that manage to work. The famous grandmother's remedies, often forgotten or little taken into account, due to their lack of scientific consistency, often give surprising results.

I would still like to mention that if you want to remedy any discomfort the most important thing is to investigate well the possible underlying causes of the disorder. Perhaps one could see if it would be possible to remove or circumscribe them. Sometimes a headache is just the consequence of a sorrow or a great disappointment that has affected us in 'our innermost being. Sometimes a hug, a smile are more effective than many medicines. The great sages of the past have often preached tolerance, humility and gratitude toward others as a system of peaceful and harmonious coexistence.

Very difficult, sometimes, to trace the causes, the real causes, that lie at the root of the problem. Often the problem stems from the mind, from the psyche, from the mysterious world of emotions. So cleaning up, relaxing, clearing the mind should be the first intervention to be done. Welcome all those activities that go in this direction: meditation, Yoga, Qi cong, singing in a choir, dancing, listening to good music, walking in the woods, donating a pinch of one's time to help others. Those who practice these things know that they are so good for the spirit and also eventually for the body. In the next book I will try to work on these things.

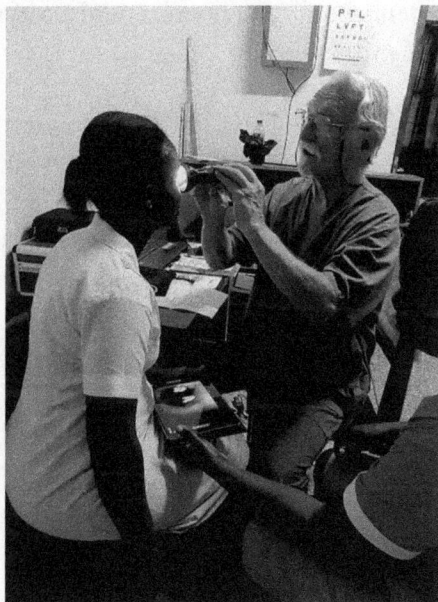

L orenzo Mazzucco was born in Florence (Italy) where he studied and started working. In the first part of his professional life he devoted himself with great passion to teaching. After graduating in Mathematics, he also taught computer science and wrote one of the first manuals to use the personal computer.

Later, he became interested in the study of holistic medicine (unconventional) and well-being in the broad sense. From shiatzu to therapeutic massage, from digito pressure to Yoga, from meditation to music and dance therapy has never stopped experimenting with different solutions to improve the state of health.

After many and varied experiences in the wellness sector in various private schools. He also studied Osteopathy and finally enrolled at the University of Florence where he obtained a degree in Podiatry which he then completed with a master's degree in Integrative Medicine.

Passionate about Traditional Chinese Medicine, he has discovered the incredible potential of Acupuncture and Auricle-therapy that have become the main activities.

Iris analysis is a particular and curious activity that has engaged him in recent times giving many gratifications.

As a volunteer he worked in a hospital in Ghana where he had incredible human and professional experiences.

BIBLIOGRAPHY

La dieta della longevità, valter longo, vallardi

I colori della salute, fabio firenzuoli, tecniche nuove

Fitoterapia, fabio firenzuoli, masson

Il piede nella medicina integrativa, lorenzo mazzucco, università di firenze

The china study, campbell,macroedizioni

Iridologia atlante illustrato e commentato, emilio ratti josef kar,l provincia autonoma di bolzano

Ansia,depressione,insonnia dall'iride, p. emilio ratti, assiri

Guarire il mal di schiena, nigel howard, armenia

Manuale di agopuntura , Peter Deadman, ea

L ' auricoloterapia, pmf nogier, librerie cortina torino

Atlante di agopuntura, hoepli

La via della leggerezza, franco berrino, daniel lumera, mondadori

Il cervello umano, asimov, bompiani

Iniziazione all'iridologia, osvaldo sponzilli, edizioni mediterranee

Conoscere l'auricoloterapia, giancarlo bazzoni, università di sassari

I fondamenti della medicina cinese, giovanni maciocia, elsevier masson

Agopuntura uno sguardo globale, franco cracolici, mind

Massaggio del piede, Wang Fu-chun, edi ermes

RINGRAZIAMENTI

Prof. Fabio Firenzuoli Università di firenze

Prof. Giancarlo Bazzoni Università di Sassari

Prof. Rudy Lanza Scuola di Naturopatia

Dott. Mario Picconi Scuola di naturopatia Panakeia

Dottor . Sonia Baccetti Centro Fior di prugna

Dott. Elisabetta Cortesi Usl Pistoia

Dott. Emilio Ratti ass.irid.italiana

www.ingramcontent.com/pod-product-compliance
Lightning Source LLC
Chambersburg PA
CBHW032055020426

42335CB00011B/352